Fetish and You
Understanding and Embracing Your Fetish

by Jackie A. Castro, MA, LMFT

Cover Layout and Design by Vinnie Corbo
Produced by Vinnie Corbo
Edited by Catherine Gigante-Brown

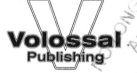

Published by Volossal Publishing
www.volossal.com

Copyright © 2014
ISBN 978-0-9909727-2-3

Table of Contents

Dedication

This book is dedicated to you, the man who courageously shared your "secret" with me. Together, we discovered that your secret was merely a sexual fetish that isn't as life-altering or as horrible as you originally imagined. The more you talked, the more you heard the fallacies of your thinking. The more you talked, the more you realized that fetish doesn't define you. The more you talked, the more relief you felt. And those therapy sessions affected change that's with you today. Thank you for allowing me to be a part of your growth.

I also want to thank each of you for speaking frankly on a topic that you've kept hidden all your life. Without your honesty and willingness to explore, I would have never been able to develop my Five-Point Fetish Plan. So, thank you for helping me to help other fetishists. I am very appreciative and eternally grateful to you.

Introduction

About five years ago, I published an article called
"You'll Never Guess What Turns Me On: Understanding Your
Sexual Fetish," and posted it on my therapy website,
www.therapywithcare.com. I have to admit that I was pleasantly
surprised at all of the attention it got. Not only did that article
receive wide acclaim, but it garnered an unprecedented amount
of emails from fetishists across the globe. They were thrilled to
come across something about fetish written from a positive,
accepting point of view.

I've long been aware that most people in the psychological
community pathologize fetish and categorize it as a paraphilia
or addiction. In short, they view it as if it's a disease instead of
a difference. There are also false claims of "cures" for fetish.
Professionals, life coaches or ministers, profess to use
behavioral conditioning techniques as a means to get the
supposed deviant "back to normal." To me, this demonstrates
a deep misunderstanding about fetish in general.

When searching online for information about sexual fetish,
it turns out that pornographers are the main supporters. While
that's great, there is a huge void for those who crave more. While
adult films provide an outlet and entertainment, fetishists are in
dire need of validation in a world that is uncompromising when
it comes to sexual expression. Especially sexual expression that
is a bit different than the perceived norm.

Perhaps you are one of these people with unusual erotic
interests. You probably feel embarrassed, alone and ashamed of
your sexual wants. You know that your arousal triggers are a bit
odd. You feel that your partner would be appalled to know what
goes on inside your head. You've tried to reprogram yourself,
only to find that you come back to your "arousal point"
(the thing that turns you on) in order to have completion during
sex. You wish your fetish would just go away. You might even
have attempted to get help, only to be disappointed. Eventually,
you go back to your one reliable source of sexual satisfaction,
to your arousal point. Hypnotherapy won't work. Conventional

12-Step Programs won't work. Most of all, abstinence won't work.

Fetish is strong, powerful and never goes away. Fetish is something that has been embedded and programmed into your sexual makeup. While there is still no definitive answer as to how fetish develops, science is now viewing fetish in much the same way it acknowledges the origins of homosexuality: it's most likely genetic.

There is an environmental factor influencing fetish as well. Early in life, a strong signal triggered a sexual response to a nonsexual stimuli. While this is interesting information, ultimately, the origin of fetish is not as important as the here and now of it is to you—the "present" that you are currently dealing with. How to make peace with your fetish and make it an integral part of your life instead of something shameful.

Many of you struggle with the secrecy aspect of having a fetish. Telling your partner. Should I or shouldn't I? You wonder if it's wrong to look at the porn that validates your cravings. You feel guilty about masturbating and thinking about your fetish. You believe that your thoughts are incorrect. You imagine that your partner would be appalled to know your real yearnings. Deep down, you feel that you are sexually broken.

Fetish and You was written to challenge your incorrect beliefs about fetish. This book will help you develop other thoughts about your sexuality: healthier, more accepting thoughts. The goal is to achieve a feeling of self-acceptance. Self-acceptance will allow you to feel confident and present in the world. Self-acceptance will give you the confidence to talk openly with your partner. And most of all, the feeling of self-acceptance will alleviate the anxiety often attached to compulsive sexual behaviors and acting out in a disordered way. Self-acceptance will also erase any feelings of self-loathing you might have.

As a licensed therapist, I have interviewed and counseled thousands of fetishists throughout my 30-year career. Embracing your fetish will enable you to manage and control your fetish. Ultimately, you want to be in control of your fetish rather than have your fetish control you.

I'm happy you have chosen to take this important journey with me.

How to Use This Book

To get the most out of *Fetish and You*, I suggest you read what I refer to as the opening chapters: those addressing what everybody should understand about any type of sexual behavior considered to be unusual by society. There are even quizzes, which I think you'll find extremely useful.

The initial chapters will give you a solid, basic foundation and understanding of what fetish is and how to deal with your emotions. You can then skip ahead to the chapter which addresses your particular sexual proclivity more specifically. I've devoted chapters to some of the most common fetishes, then have a "catch-all" chapter called "The Less-Common Fetishes: Off the Beaten Track," which discusses the brand of fetish that is more specialized. If your particular fetish is not included, please don't be discouraged or disappointed. The chapter called "Identification" gives you the questions you must ask yourself in order to complete the Identification Process. You can then choose one of the chapters that deals with a specific fetish and use that as a model to help you understand your own fetish.

And finally, there are "wrap-up" chapters which discuss key topics like managing your fetish, whether or not you should share your fetish with your partner, case studies and how to successfully incorporate fetish into your life. These chapters are intended for everyone to read, no matter their personal proclivity.

I've often said that fetishes are as different as fingerprints or snowflakes. Because of this, it's impossible to address them all in a book. However, I've provided general guidelines on addressing and accepting your particular fetish, no matter how "deviant" and "perverted" our closed culture has made you out to be. You are in a safe place now—no judgment, no name-calling, no finger-pointing. Just useful information and acceptance.

Let's move forward together.

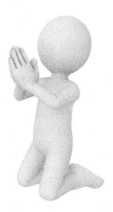

Chapter 1 - Our Puritanical Society

We live in a world that loves to assign labels. This is the way we categorize people, places and things. But all too often, these labels are rigid, unyielding and leave little room for variation. We're smart or stupid. Tall or short. Happy or sad. We form opinions about others based upon what we were told as children. These opinions are often racially based and full of stereotypes. Yet, because we've heard these things during our formative years, we think of them as the Gospel truth. We don't question what we're told. We just formulate incorrect belief systems which we adopt and adapt as our own. We don't even think to question the facts.

Gender dictates a great deal of how we view the world, as well as how we see ourselves. From the moment we're born, we're expected to behave in accordance with being male or female. Pink or blue. Ballet or sports. English or math. Think about all the differences we take for granted simply based upon gender. Parents treat girl babies differently than boy babies. Girls are handled daintily while boys are roughhoused. Girls are expected to be well-behaved while boys are given more leeway, often with the shrug, "Boys will be boys." But what exactly does that mean?

Though much progress has been made, these societal standards still exist. By and large, men are expected to be the main financial supporters of their family. Women can work outside the house, but it's not required. Men statistically earn more money for the same job. Eyebrows are still raised if a man chooses to be a stay-at-home dad while his wife goes out to bring home the bacon. Things are definitely changing but double standards still exist. Women are still thought of as emotionally driven while men are portrayed as rational decision makers.

An interesting case to prove this point came about during the 2004 presidential primaries. We had two very controversial candidates to choose from—an African-American male and a Caucasian female. Both of these candidates crossed cultural norms and challenged racially-driven attitudes. When push came to shove, the African-American male triumphed over the Caucasian female. Of course, there were many other factors present, but think about the outcome. Even in our "progressive" country, we still consider women to be second class by the very nature of their sex. Yes, we've evolved, but we still have a long way to go toward genuine equality between men and women.

Along with these messages about sexual gender come even stronger messages about how to express our sexual behavior. Universally, girls are taught that their sexuality is something to be protected. Sex can be a useful tool in solidifying a relationship, controlling a partner and, of course, creating life. Boys are given a completely different message. They are encouraged to explore, conquer, and get as much as possible. Boys are schooled to be careful about making babies but the other messages seem to hold more importance. Promiscuous boys are players while promiscuous girls are sluts. Guys are expected to be initiators while girls who take the lead are labeled as aggressive. Suffice to say that there's a huge difference when it comes to the expectations the world community bestows on us simply by the virtue of being born male or female.

Sex is a topic that human beings don't really like to discuss. Parents dread questions about sex from their kids. These days, moms and dads are happy (and relieved!) that most schools offer basic sex education. But the information given is generally awkward and often unconvincing. When it comes to sex talk, it's universally met with embarrassment, shame and a touch of childish snickering. As a result, we embrace inflexible beliefs that validate the concept of "normalcy." We fall back upon stereotypes and myths that have been handed down from generation to generation.

There are scores of rigid sexual beliefs that go something like this:

- Sex should be performed between one man and one woman.
- Sex means that the male inserts his penis into the woman's vagina. This is called intercourse.
- Intercourse should be performed between a man and woman who are in love and better yet, married.
- Intercourse also produces babies. Some religions advocate sex only for the purpose of procreation.
- Men are the initiators when it comes to sex.
- Men are the aggressors in matters sexual.
- Women submit to the sexual act upon her man's desires.
- Ejaculation is the goal and completes the act of intercourse.

Within the last four decades, thanks to sexologists like Masters and Johnson, we've broadened our views to include gems like this:

- Women have a clitoris, which is instrumental in female sexual pleasure.
- Women have orgasms from either intercourse or clitoral stimulation.
- It's okay, and even preferable, for a woman to enjoy sex.
- Men can perform cunnilingus and still be considered "men."
- Marital aids or sex toys like vibrators are fine to incorporate into the sex act.
- Some kinky play like light bondage or teasing with feathers is acceptable.

We have definitely made immense strides in our knowledge about sexuality, but our core beliefs are far from progressive. The letters LGBT (which stand for "lesbian, gay, bisexual and transgender") are as common as USA or LOL. But deep down, we're not as accepting as we pretend to be. Awareness is a totally different beast than genuine acceptance. Lesbians are still seen as women who have "settled" for a female because they are masculine, inferior or hurt. Gay men are sissies and not real men. Bisexuals are thought of as mainly gay or just plain horny. And transgenders are still a mystery to just about everyone. The very idea of the sex-change process is still considered pretty abhorrent

Although many US states sanction gay marriage, I'm referring to society's general belief system rather than legalities. People will give lip service to the LGBT community but if they were totally honest, most parents pray for a straight child. The negative messages are so ingrained that many LGBT people keep their sexual preference a secret from their family and at their job. Is the world really more open-minded? Are we changing our old, antiquated beliefs? Maybe a little, but we still have a long way to go.

Science is discovering that people do not choose to be gay, straight or transgender. Today there is evidence that sexuality is genetically preordained. Human beings are born with their sexual map in place. Nobody chooses to be straight or gay. And we don't choose our predilections either. This includes you, the forgotten population. You, the man who has a sexual fetish. There, I said it.

You didn't choose to have a fetish. Your fetish chose you. And just like the LGBT population, you too must contend with a population that is unyielding and rigid about any kind of sexuality that is different from the norm. But unlike those in the LGBT population, you have to deal with something even more insidious. Loneliness.

The idea of sexual fetish is relatively new. Many of you probably didn't even know how to define the fact that your penis gets erect when exposed to thoughts or stimuli different than what you were schooled to think was arousing. Remember, sex education is rudimentary. It covers only the basics. Chances are good that no one ever mentioned the fact that hundreds of thousands of you (maybe more) get aroused by words, objects and acts outside the confines of conventional sexuality.

Many of you have been helped by the Internet. Finally, you know that you aren't alone. But a large number of you have been dealing with your fetish since the pre-Internet days. I know how you've suffered. I know how you've felt so plagued and disgusted with yourself. No matter how many websites profess to specialize in your fetish, if you were completely honest with yourself, you still feel isolated and alone. You believe there is something "wrong" with you. No woman will want you. You envy the LGBT community for their openness and support system. You wish there was a community of fetishists. (Actually, there is. Many large cities like New York have fetish "clubs" like the Eulenspiegel Society or TES, http://www.tes.org/ and fetlife.com) Unfortunately, this self-loathing keeps everyone apart. We don't want the stigma of being sexually different. Especially when it's something we conceive to be embarrassing and perverse.

I realize that many of you feel you're condemned to live a life without intimacy, especially within the confines of a sexually-inflexible global community. How in the world are you going to explain that you'd rather suck your lover's toes than her nipples? How can you tell your wife that you'd rather see her dressed in thigh-high boots than in a negligee? That your need for pain is stronger than your need for pleasure?

Your dilemma is not unfounded. Nor are your feelings of confusion, shame and guilt. How do you expect to function normally in a culture where there are so many predisposed expectations about sex, relationships and male/female roles? No wonder you live in a constant state of anxiety and fear about your fetish! No wonder you're baffled about how to have your fetish and a relationship, too. Your concern is completely understandable considering that we live in a world filled with prejudice.

But there is hope.

The good news is that people are beginning to acknowledge that fetish or offbeat sexuality does in fact exist. Years ago people equated bondage and discipline with severe, dark sadomasochistic behavior. Today sex shops sell user-friendly kits that incorporate aspects of these behaviors without the grit—or guilt. It's no big deal to restrain your partner with silk scarves and use soft feathers and floggers to tease and torment. Leather and latex events are held in major cities across the US and

Europe. The book *Fifty Shades of Grey* was a blockbuster, enjoyed by conventional housewives across the globe, and the film based on the novel promises to be just as successful.

The Internet is filled with websites that cater to every conceivable fetish. And new ones are emerging all the time. Furries (people who enjoy dressing up like furry animals) are common with the younger crowd. I suspect the furry phenomenon occurred because of the cuddly, larger-than-life characters kids were exposed to at amusement parks. There's also something called "cake farts," where a person plops down onto a cake and passes gas. There are "casting" fetishists who enjoy being out in public with casts covering their make-believe broken arms and legs. And there are all kinds of fetishes inspired by body piercings and tattoos.

Like some sports, these fetishes often go to the extreme. They are reflective of the times. Best of all, they embrace the uniqueness of the human condition. They are the embodiment of the catch phrase "Let your freak flag fly."

As an advocate for fetishists for more than three decades, I've seen attitudes grow, develop and change. I've worked with women who are open-minded and want to do whatever it takes to be their husband's best lover. They totally "get" the notion that having intimate knowledge of their man's fetish is the secret to turning him on.

Yet, I know that you still have serious doubts about acceptance from another human being, especially one you care about. But here's the good news—it all starts with you. You have the power to change your thinking. You have the power to manage your fetish. Your fetish doesn't cause your negativity— you do. The shame and guilt you feel are only there because of how you think and the fact that you've bought into rigid, uncompromising beliefs.

I will guarantee you this—the more you feel okay about your fetish, the less anxious you will feel. The less anxious you feel, the less importance you will give your fetish. You will acknowledge its existence and put it in the right perspective. You will know that the fetish defines only one small part of you. You are, in fact, a human being with potential to contribute to the world, your family and the community in the best way possible.

You have all of the assets, abilities and personality traits which allow you to be uniquely YOU. Fetish is but a small part of who you are.

Once you reach this transformative phase of self-acceptance, you will have achieved the basic component of what it takes to feel comfortable with your fetish, to peacefully coexist with it. But first, some education. It's important to know what fetish really means. That's what we'll look at in the next chapter.

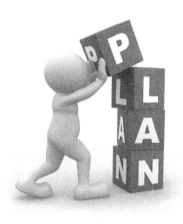

Chapter 2 – The Five-Point Fetish Plan

If you are a male who has unconventional sexual longings, this book is meant for you. Unconventional means that you are aroused by a specific object, activity or mindset that's generally not related to typical sexual activity. This arousal trigger, also known as fetish, is necessary in order for you to achieve orgasm. These arousal triggers are not connected with standard heterosexual behavior. Although they are different, they are very real for you.

Though women and people in the LGBT community also have fetishes, for the sake of simplicity, the focus of this book is from the heterosexual male point of view. If you are female or someone in the LGBT community, please mentally switch the pronouns. I'm confident that you will learn from *Fetish and You* as much as your male counterpart will. I'm a staunch advocate for all people who have a sexual fetish. You are an extremely misunderstood group and it's time for you to have a voice and be heard.

If you are a male, young or old, married or single, chances are good that your sexual preference has caused turmoil and struggle in your life. You struggle because you have shame. You struggle because you feel guilty when indulging your fetish. Your major relief is masturbating to fetish pornography, but then you feel bad about yourself for doing so. Most sex therapists will tell you that you can stop and that you have a sexual addiction. I am not one of those therapists. I don't believe this is true. I believe that you have a fetish that can be managed, controlled and effectively incorporated into your life.

By the end of this book, you will understand what fetish is all about, plus you'll come to a place of reckoning, identify the components of your unique fetish and ultimately make a thoughtful decision about how to blend fetish into your life in a way that makes sense for you. I've come up with an easy *Five-Point Fetish Plan* that will give you tools to manage your own particular fetish.

1. Understanding Fetish (Chapters 3 & 4)

Did you know that most people who have a fetish have no idea what fetish is? That makes sense because most of you have had this "quirk" all of your lives. From the moment you had your first orgasm, you probably recall that you were triggered by some thing, some words, or some body part that you knew was a little offbeat.

You probably thought nothing of it at the time. However, once you passed puberty and became a full-fledged sexual being, you probably noticed that something was different about you. You probably tried to fight the feeling. Some of you were able to form conventional relationships with women but your fetish came to mind when you were alone. Others have a stronger demand. Those of you must have some kind of fetish "event" present in order to be sexually fulfilled. And as time progresses, this demand has now become problematic.

Congratulations. You finally found a name for what you have. You figured out that you have a sexual fetish. But what is that anyway? It's necessary to know what sexual fetish means before you can accept it. In other words, you can't accept what you don't understand. I am committed to helping you understand your fetish.

2. Accepting Your Fetish (Chapters 5 & 6)

Self-acceptance is key in order for you to healthfully incorporate fetish into your life. Right now, you probably have anxiety about your fetish. That's because you feel different than your male peers. As a result, you feel shame. You feel like something's wrong with you. Even worse, you blame yourself. As a result, you try not to "feed" your fetish. You stay away from magazines, DVDs and websites. Yet, eventually you can't help yourself. You reluctantly give into your yearnings. You have sex or masturbate. The fetish image comes into your head at the moment of orgasm.

After you climax, you feel angry and ashamed of your "weakness." You feel bad about yourself. So, you start to masturbate again in an attempt to feel better. You get downhearted and depressed. You feel hopeless. The shame cycle begins.

Gaining a sense of self-compassion is the only way to combat the darkness of shame, remorse and guilt. The more accepting you are, the less anxious you feel. As a result, you won't feel so sexually hungry. You'll have a sense of serenity knowing that your needs will be met. The inner turmoil subsides. You'll be at peace with your fetish. Best of all, you'll be able to proceed with your life! It's my goal to get you to accept your fetish and yourself.

3. Identifying the Components of Your Fetish (Chapters 7-15)

It's not enough to name your fetish—you must know the details. Identification will show you how to create a comprehensive inventory of your fetish requirements. This process will enable you to have a definitive idea of what fetish fulfillment means to you. You must know yourself before you can hope to have anyone else know you. Identification provides the blueprint in order to effectively communicate to another person.

If you don't fully understand your fetish, no one else will either. Even the most experienced professional fantasy fulfiller has to know more than generalities about your fetish. They'll have know what words you like to hear, what costumes you'd like to see, and the sensations you'd like to feel—the tiny details that only you recognize because they are unique to you. No one is a mind reader and every fetishist is distinct. Identification gives you the opportunity to be the definitive expert on your fetish wishes as well as your desires. I'll assist you in identifying the integral parts of your fetish.

4. Communicating about Your Fetish (Chapters 16-18)

Acceptance and identification are necessary steps before you even think about sharing your fetish with another person. Once you complete your Identification Process, you'll be ready to make an important decision. Do you want to share your fetish with another person? If so, with whom? Your wife? Your lover? Another fetishist? A professional Dominatrix?

Before you jump in and eagerly blurt out your innermost secrets to someone else, take pause. Communication is a skill that must be learned and developed. Talking about your fetish just might be the single most challenging message you'll ever convey. Take a moment to learn some basic communication techniques — and hone them.

In order to effectively communicate, you must be confident, knowledgeable and know what you're going to say. This is why you have to work through your burdensome feelings of shame and guilt before you ever attempt to talk about fetish. It's very difficult to speak about something when you're still experiencing inner turmoil. Once you achieve inner peace, you'll be able to think more clearly about your fetish. That's why self-acceptance is so vital. In many ways, self-acceptance is the most important aspect of this entire program. Without it, you will always be struggling.

The ultimate purpose of communication is to help another human being understand you better. And, if you are communicating to a partner whom you'll be interacting with, you'll need to be able to talk about every last detail of your fetish. The more you communicate, the better your experience will be. I'll usher you through this aspect.

5. Managing and Incorporating Fetish into Your Life (Chapters 19-22)

You are the captain of your ship. Your life belongs to you. And likewise, you control your fetish; your fetish does not control you. With that being said, how can you find a place for fetish in your life? How do you address your fetish necessities in a healthy, balanced and holistic way?

When you come from a place of inner peace, you will be able to make a rational decision. You'll have a good idea about what realistically will work for you. Fetish is no longer a secret you keep from your partner—unless you elect to have it be your solitary pleasure. Fetish is no longer shameful. It's simply a part of your sexual makeup. It's part of who you are. Notice that I said "part of," not "all of" who you are. It's just an aspect of you, like your profession or your political affiliation.

To recap, fetish is merely a quirk you were born with. It does not make you good or bad. It does not make you healthy or unhealthy. It's but one small element that makes up the pieces that are "you." It's solely your choice whether or not to make it a part of your life in whatever manner you choose, and in whatever way works best for you.

In Summary

The *Five-Point Fetish Plan* is time-tested and it works. I've used it repeatedly with the individuals who come to me for counseling. Fetishists who do the work diligently get excellent results. With dedication and effort, you'll get good results, too. Just be patent and kind to yourself. Change doesn't happen overnight.

Remember that you weren't born feeling shameful and guilty. Your belief system took years to develop. It was shaped through the teachings of your parents, educators and society. Because these ideas are so ingrained in your being, give yourself time to redevelop your old ideas and thoughts.

This book isn't meant to be read from start to finish in one sitting. Following the *Five-Point Fetish Plan* takes a great deal of consideration and introspection. You must give yourself the space to be thoughtful, the time to write, and think some more. You owe it to yourself to thoroughly learn how to accept a part of yourself that needs guidance and nurturing.

It's time to be free. It's time to start living. And that means living, embracing and enjoying your fetish.

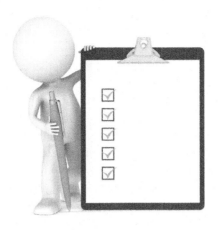

Chapter 3 - Fetish Quiz:
What's Your Fetish Sensibility?

Fetish is a word that is now finding its way into our everyday speech. We used to think of fetish as something mysterious, dark and a little foreboding. But these days the word is colloquial and everyday. People say they have a "fetish" for ice cream or a "cleaning fetish." Adult bookstores even sell "fetish kits" which contain things like light restraints, whips and feathers.

While the world appears to be more open to "kink," the general public's mindset is as closed as ever. There's still a grave misunderstanding about the kind of fetish that's deeply ingrained...like your fetish, for instance. The kind of fetish that rules your masturbatory fantasies and drives you to orgasm. The fetish that's been with you ever since you were born and mostly likely will be with you the rest of your life.

Sexual fetish is not a preference. It's a need. A fetish is something very specific that turns you on so much that it's almost painful. When you come in contact with or see a fetish image, you feel an overwhelming sense of lust. It feels both good and bad. Good in the fact that you are hyper-stimulated; bad because you can't get your desires met in the moment. It's like being locked in a strip club. You can look but you can't release. A fetishist feels this frustration all the time. Depending on your fetish, you are often bombarded with reminders of your fetish everywhere you turn.

Early on, you didn't understand your fetish completely. You only understood that certain body parts, articles of clothing or fabrics made you feel "funny" or even uncomfortable inside. It wasn't until you hit puberty that you realized the mere thought of your fetish triggered an erection. As you became more sexual, you made the connection. Today, you realize that some kind of fetish image is necessary in order for you to orgasm. This realization is a blessing and a curse. You're blessed because you have a fantasy that will reliably turn you on enough to orgasm. You're cursed because you feel different than other men. Cursed because you question your sanity, and sometimes, even worse.

Always remember that you didn't choose your fetish. It chose you. You might have a vague idea of where it came from. Or you have no idea of how you made the connection. All you know is that your fetish cravings carry great magnitude. They are ever-present. Some days the "itch" is stronger than others. You have no clue why your interest continues to grow, yet it does. Sometimes it seems like you can't help but indulge, and you do. Sometimes grudgingly and guiltily, and other times with an insatiable hunger. The Internet makes life easy because satisfaction is just a click away. Your fetish is probably the first thing you ever Googled.

Fetish is strong, powerful and never goes away. Your fetish never disappears, no matter how much you wish it would. No matter how much you'd like to be the same as everyone else. The funny part is that your next-door neighbor, your boss or even your best friend might also have a fetish. How would you know? Fetish is everyone's "dirty little secret."

But hand in hand with the secrets, come shame and guilt. If the fetish is wrong, it means that you're wrong, too. You hide the fetish the way you'd hide a crime you got away with—you spend part of each day wondering if you're going to get "caught." The shame drives you to be secretive. The secrets lead to paralyzing guilt. Human beings are not equipped to hide big truths from our significant others in their lives. In time, we're left feeling profoundly lonely.

Ultimately, you believe that your fetish makes you inferior. Less than a man. Unlovable. You feel separate and distant from others. You think that no one understands. And in a way, you're right. At this point, you barely understand fetish yourself. How then, can you possibly communicate the minutiae of your fetish to another human being?

No woman would want you if she knew. You are convinced that something is wrong with you. You think that women will reject you based on your fetish needs. Having these negative thoughts are common to almost every fetishist.

Before we delve in any further, please take the quiz below to test your fetish perception. Jot down your responses on a sheet of paper so you can check your score. How many of these thoughts have you had?

Fetish Quiz # 1 – Your Fetish Perception:
1. My fetish makes me a freak.
2. My fetish is sick and perverse.
3. I'll keep my fetish a secret until the day I die.
4. I'm not a good person because I have a fetish.
5. I hate that I have a fetish.
6. No woman would want me if they knew what I really desire.
7. It's completely wrong that I think of fetish in order to have an orgasm.
8. Fighting my fetish makes me feel that there's hope for me. Maybe I'll be forgiven on Judgment Day.
9. I'll never accept this part of myself.
10. I'm nothing but an addict.

How to Score
If you related to even one of these statements, you're in the right place. If you related to three or more, you definitely will benefit from the help and guidance this book offers. In truth, most fetishists who haven't received guidance and education probably relate to every single one of the above statements.

These types of thoughts are self-deprecating and unhelpful. They do not allow you to be who you are. They leave you feeling stuck and hopeless.

A Taste of What's To Come

Let's look at some of the thoughts of an evolved fetishist. How many of these do you believe right now? How many of them would you like to adapt as your own?

Fetish Quiz # 2 – An Evolved Fetishist's Perception:

1. My fetish means that I have "out-of-the-box" proclivities.
2. My fetish is a little quirky, but it's just one part of my sexuality.
3. My fetish is sexually based. The only person who ever has to know is my partner. Even, then, disclosure is solely my choice.
4. I'm a good person based upon my behaviors, interactions and values. Fetish has no bearing on my character.
5. I accept that I have a fetish.
6. I am respectful of the fact that my partner or future partner may not initially understand my fetish. I can make a mindful decision about whether or not I want to tell my partner about my fetish.
7. My thoughts can never hurt anyone. I'm lucky to have something to think about that reliably helps me to orgasm.
8. I don't believe I'll be judged based on my fetish. By accepting myself, I can use my energy to be the best person I can be.
9. The more I learn, the more I know that I'm okay.
10. I'm in control of my fetish. It doesn't control me. I incorporate fetish into my life in a safe, sane, balanced way.

How to Score

How many of the modified statements did you agree with? If you agreed even once, you have an open mind. It's my hope that by the end of this book, you'll not only agree with every statement but that you will be living every statement.

If you follow the guidelines in this book, in time you'll be able to internalize these 10 empowering statements into your own personal beliefs system.

Discard your old ideas and adapt these new ones. Look carefully at the evolved fetishist's modified beliefs. You'll notice that they are more rationally based. They are nonjudgmental and factual. This is in contrast to your original ideas that are emotionally based, critical and self-deprecating.

Please feel free to add your own statements to either list. What are some of your present ideas? How would you like to think once you are finished with this program?

In Summary

Having a fetish doesn't mean condemning yourself to a life of shame with a side order of anxiety. Instead, it's in your power to understand, accept and enjoy your fetish.

You can adapt a more evolved way of thinking. This new way of thinking will foster change in your beliefs about fetish. These new ideas will alter the way you interact with yourself and those around you. Your positive attitude will be evident. So will your self-confidence. Be assured that good things await.

Let's get ready to do the work!

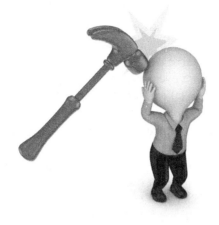

Chapter 4 - Understanding Fetish and the Impact It Has on You

Imagine that we were all destined to live a life that was preordained. Imagine that we were only allowed to enjoy one kind of food, one place for vacation and one form of recreation. That we were told how many children we could have, that we were given only one career option and our life partner was prearranged. Imagine a life of no choice or decision. Our very existence would be mundane, boring and joyless.

As humans we are blessed with intellect, reason and a certain amount of freedom. However, when it comes to human sexuality, freedom is not generally embraced by the social order. Our thinking about sexuality is extremely rigid and most people are educated to believe that heterosexual sex is the most acceptable form of interaction. While we tolerate some variables, the original ideas about sex remain the same. One man. One woman. Preferably married and engaging in intercourse with some foreplay approximately three times per week. That's the norm. And that's what we strive to achieve.

Yet, the reality about sex is that it's as varied as the human race. Every person on this planet has something which is uniquely "theirs" when it comes to sex. One particular spot on your body that responds well to touch. One smell that is arousing. A sound or phrase that puts you over the edge. Everyone is distinctive when it comes to sexual preference and taste. That's why we eventually find that one person who meets our sexual needs. It takes some looking but we usually find them.

But sometimes this person is harder to find because our sexual preferences are a bit unusual and we don't understand exactly what we want or require.

Let's begin by figuring out fetish. Education is your first step in understanding your own particular yen and getting your needs met.

How is sexual fetish defined?

In plain language, people who have a fetish, sexualize something as opposed to someone. That "something" may be an object, an act or a behavior. The fetish can involve the use of nonliving objects such as panties, a cigarette or an angora sweater. The fetish can also be a fixation on a certain part of the body such as feet, the buttocks or lips. Some like to enjoy the body part in a particular state, such as hairy armpits, long finger nails painted red or feet that are unwashed. Some fetishists enjoy hearing certain words, phrases or statements. Others like specific acts such as trampling, smothering or whipping. These acts can be stand-alone activities for some, or incorporated into a role-play situation.

The important aspect to note is that fetish is something that's extremely specific and well-defined. A fetishist has very particular desires that are not generally associated with conventional sex yet provide arousal and release in a sexual manner.

I've said it before and I'll say it again: fetish is strong, powerful and never goes away. (Perhaps this should be your mantra.)

Fetish is a part of your sexual makeup and has been with you all your life. Many of you can probably trace it back as early as age five. Most of the time it lays dormant during the latency phase of our lives, but it re-emerges once we become sexual beings.

Fetish is the major thing that gets your juices going. If you were to pick one sex act and no others, most of you would choose your fetish over conventional sex. This doesn't make you wrong or bad. It simply acknowledges who you are and how strongly fetish needs are ingrained. Many of you have tried to will away your fetish, concentrate on other sexual activities and pretend your fetish doesn't exist. But it always returns with a vengeance, doesn't it? This is no reflection on you and certainly doesn't make you weak. It's simply the nature of fetish. You can't turn a gay man straight and you can't make a fetish go away.

Where does fetish come from?

The etiology, or cause, of fetishism is not recognized conclusively. This is to say that many in the professional community believe a variety of theories about the origin of fetish. One current school of thought supports the belief that fetish has physiological causal—that it's associated with abnormalities in the brain's temporal lobe. In other words, you are born with the fetish gene. However, environmental factors must be present in order to activate the growth of fetish. These environmental factors are associated with imprinting, meaning that something impacted you very, very early in life which then was added to your arousal template.

For example, if you get aroused by smothering, perhaps you played wrestling games when you were younger and a playmate sat on your face. Or, if you are aroused by paddling, perhaps you were threatened with or heard about paddling in a school which permitted corporal punishment.

Fear, excitement, and curiosity are powerful emotions. When we experience them, the body remembers the charge they gave us physiologically, and for some of us, those moments become eroticized on a subconscious level. This even includes scary childhood moments like spanking. In response, we protected ourselves by sexualizing these powerful feelings. Generally, these feelings lay dormant until we become sexually active. Then, out of nowhere, we connect our original moment of excitement and experience with a powerful erotic charge. This feeling is so strong that our sexuality is linked to this early sexual/excitement/fear moment.

These potent emotions linked to the fetish are stored in the subconscious mind. They are connected to a part of our brain that produces sexual stimulation. When puberty strikes, these thoughts and feelings re-emerge. Before we realize what's happening, we are associating our childhood fear/excitement to adult sexual feelings.

The environmental factors and early triggers aspect of fetish make a great deal of sense. But right now, you're probably wondering, "Why me?" A lot of kids playfully wrestle with each other when they're younger, but when they grow up, they don't want their girlfriends to sit on their faces for the purpose of smothering. Many children are spanked or paddled but most of them don't want to think about those awful memories, let alone re-experience them erotically as adults.

Scientific research on fetish is similar to the current school of thought on homosexuality, and even addiction. No one really chooses their sexuality or compulsive behaviors. Environmental conditions allow these predisposed tendencies to bloom and fester.

Prior to more recent scientific studies, Sigmund Freud suggested that fetishism is a learned behavior that results when a normal sexual stimulus is paired with a fetish item. Here are a few examples:

> A male toddler crawls on the floor. Inadvertently, his penis rubs against his mother's shoe. The resulting pleasure is then associated with the shoe, and a foot fetish is likely to develop.

> A boy is subjected to a "wedgie" on the school playground when a group of his friends grabbed his underwear and pulled them up so hard that the material was caught between his buttock cheeks. The boy feels embarrassed and humiliated, but at the same time, his penis is stimulated. As a result, a connection is made between a wedgie and sexual excitement.

A boy visits his friend who has a pretty, older sister.
She leaves her underwear to dry on top of the washing
machine. The boy is curious and touches the panties.
An arousal occurs and later, there is a strong
association between the feel of women's underwear
and sexual arousal.

There are clearly environmental links between charged
experiences that happened early in life and fetishism. Today,
psychology still acknowledges environmental factors but also
includes genetic predispositions. That's why everyone who has
an experience like this doesn't develop a fetish. But as for you...
you already had the gene. Whatever happened early on activated
the predisposed fetishistic response. Does that make sense?
I hope it does and that it gives your fetish some validation.

When did you first discover that you had a proclivity toward your fetish?

Most people have memories about their fetish from very
early on. Many report feeling "funny" or having "butterflies
in their stomach" (or that "butterfly" feeling in their genitals)
as early as four or six years of age. Usually these feelings lay
dormant during the latency period and re-emerge during puberty.
At that time, something accidental occurs, that re-triggers the
original arousal.

Sometimes the fetish is prompted by a scene in a movie or by
being in contact with the object, such as a woman wearing
stiletto heels, high-cut boots or leather. The feeling of arousal
is undeniable during these moments and the fetishist is then
encouraged to explore further. With the advent of the Internet,
fetish material is easily accessible, only a click away.

Do you find yourself thinking about your fetish often?

Once one discovers their fetish, it's very similar to the
phenomenon of discovering sex. There's a lot of curiosity,
feelings of arousal and a craving for satisfaction. Often, when
a teenager learns about sex, they can think of nothing else. It's
similar with a fetish.

Again, most fetishists get many of their needs fulfilled online. They might be drawn to indulge in viewing images of their fetish every time they're on the computer and fight the yearnings. But the more they deny their desires, the stronger these desires become. Because of this withholding, the "itch" becomes stronger and stronger until they give in, and then they often feel badly about their "weakness."

Do you have a strong connection to your fetish with orgasm?

Whatever the fetish, it's your point of arousal. Many people who have a fetish do not act upon their fetish. Instead of receiving fulfillment with another human being, they go online and view fetishistic images in order to facilitate with masturbation. However, masturbation is necessary in order to validate the real source of arousal—the fetish.

Indulging in fetishistic thoughts might be the only time you feel that you're being honest about what really turns you on. Therefore, it feels particularly wonderful to orgasm while masturbating at the time you're connected to your favorite adult website. This is because you're being totally free and truthful with yourself when you acknowledge your fetish and masturbate. You're unencumbered by self-doubt and self-judgment.

Understanding Offbeat Sexuality

The technical terminology is less important than the reality of the definition of what "out of the norm" sexuality means to you. If you want to be correct and precise, your behavior falls under the category of "sexual paraphilia" with a subcategory of sexual fetish, thrown in for good measure. But personally, I feel it's more helpful and healing to think of your sexuality as being offbeat, progressive and best of all, avant-garde.

Take a look at the definition of avant-garde. Basically, it means to represent a pushing of the boundaries of what is accepted as the norm or the status quo, primarily in the cultural realm. It can also be used to refer to people or works that are experimental and innovative, particularly with respect to art, culture and politics. Now, that's not so bad is it? We're merely extending the definition of avant-garde to include sexuality.

Is Fetish Harmful or Dangerous?

First and foremost, please don't confuse fetish with addiction. A fetish is not an addiction. It simply defines your point of arousal. The only time a fetish can be harmful, addictive or disordered is when the fetish becomes all-consuming or compulsive. Often, fetishists feel so bad about being sexually different, that they develop anxiety. When anxiety takes over, so does a need to self-soothe and distract. The fetish then becomes a reliable way to emotionally self-regulate and a vicious cycle gets established, which can sometimes manifest itself like this:

> You feel anxious, so you visit your favorite fetish
> website and masturbate to orgasm. You then feel guilty
> for doing so. The guilt morphs into a sense of uncertainty
> about the fetish. This causes you to feel even more
> anxious, so you masturbate again. Now you feel even
> worse. You start thinking that something is seriously
> wrong with you and that you are terribly alone. In an
> attempt not to feel so isolated, you go to yet another
> website which proves there are others out there in
> cyberspace like you. Since you still want to feel better,
> you decide to masturbate for a third time. As soon you
> orgasm, you might feel bad about yourself once more,
> and once more, your fears about yourself and your fetish
> are validated. And there's that dark sense of dread that
> you are a lonely freak.
>
> See how this gets going?

Throughout my career as a therapist, I've observed a huge link between anxiety and fetish. Once you understand that fetish is actually your own personal norm, you'll feel less anxious. With less anxiety, you'll have less of a inclination to soothe yourself—and most likely, you'll masturbate less obsessively. What's more, you'll accept your fetish and understand that it's here to stay. As a result, you will experience a sense of peace about your fetish. With peace, your anxiety diminishes and you can focus in on other aspects of your life. The compulsive behaviors will ease and your impulse to self-soothe will not be so prevalent.

In time, you might even come to a place of embracement. You will learn to not only accept, but also, to enjoy your fetish. Think of it this way: Most people get bored with conventional sex. This means that their sexual feelings wane over time. Not true of fetishists. I've seen fetishists well into their 80s who remain aroused and engaged when thinking about or participating in fetish activities. With a fetish you will always have a reliable way to feel sexually aroused. Isn't that cool?

So, you see, your fetish is far from being a curse. It can actually be considered a blessing, something to honor about yourself. You can begin to think of yourself as being one of the lucky ones!

Other Characteristics of the Fetishist: Which of these do you identify with?
1. I think of my fetish when I'm not having sex.
2. I think of my fetish in order to get myself turned on prior to sex.
3. I think of my fetish during sex.
4. I think of my fetish when I'm having an orgasm.
5. I visit fetish websites.
6. I want to talk about fetish to the women I date but I wouldn't dare.
7. I'd like to find someone who would accept my fetish and participate in it with me but I doubt this kind of woman exists.
8. When I think of my fetish I experience feelings of shame.
9. I wish I could get rid of my fetish desires.
10. I believe my fetish makes me a perverted human being.
11. I often want to engage fetish-wise with non-consenting adults even though I know it's wrong.
12. I believe fetish is getting in the way of my living a good life.
13. I'm pretty sure that if my wife or girlfriend knew about my fetish, she'd leave me.
14. I believe that having a fetish would be a deal-breaker for most women.
15. My religious beliefs conflict with my fetish desires.
16. I believe I'll go to hell because of my fetish.

17. I try hard to suppress my fetish desires.
18. I am ashamed and embarrassed of my fetish.
19. I try to suppress my fetish desires.
20. I am ashamed and embarrased of my fetish.

Most of you will identify with some, if not a number of, the above statements. I've talked to thousands of fetishists throughout my extensive career. All of them have spoken of the intense discomfort associated with fetish. All of them have wished it would go away.

Years ago, I ran support groups for people who had fetishes. I'd often pose the question, "If I could give you a pill that would erase your fetish forever, would you take it?" Most participants raised their hands without question. They all felt horribly uncomfortable with having a penchant for sexual wants out of the norm.

Well, I have good news and bad news for you. The bad news is that I don't have that pill and I don't believe there is a cure for your fetish. But the good news is that I can help you to get rid of each of those 20 thoughts listed above. I can get you to reformulate your old ideas and beliefs about fetish. In time, you may even describe yourself as someone who has offbeat, quirky or evolved sexual desires.

When you reach that point, the word "fetish" might be too clinical or generalized for you. That's because you will think of yourself as a cool, multifaceted individual with adventurous sexual proclivities. Sounds pretty good, doesn't it? And that, my friend, describes you to a T. You are that cool guy with a taste for the unusual. My goal is to prove it to you.

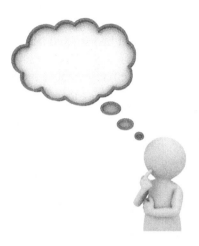

Chapter 5 - Think Your Way to Acceptance

Most of you think your "problem" is that you have a fetish. But here's the real truth: Your issue is not that you have a fetish but how you perceive your fetish.

Clinical research has proven that our moods are directly related to our thoughts. Modern psychology has adapted an evidence-based theory that proves there is a causal link between thinking and feeling. If we fail a test and feel ashamed, most likely we are admonishing ourselves for not studying harder and calling ourselves names like loser, lazy or stupid. When we are faced with a new situation and feel anxious, we are most likely telling ourselves that no one will like us, we're not capable or we will fail the task. When we wake up and feel depressed, we think discouraging thoughts. We tell ourselves that our lives are going nowhere, nothing will ever change and that there's ultimately no point in doing whatever we're doing.

Even if we are not consciously aware of these thoughts, they are still there, chipping away at our psyche. Think of a time when you were feeling unhappy or anxious. What were you telling yourself in the moment? If I photographed you in that instant, what would be the caption beneath the picture? Most likely, it would be some kind of statement that would be reflective of the way you were feeling. Thoughts like, "Everyone else has it better," or "If only I had studied harder in school," and "I should never have done that." Do you see how each of the above statements can produce feelings of sadness, regret, anger and guilt?

These negatively-based thoughts almost always have flaws. They are not based on fact. They are not rational. We call ourselves names. We make predictions about situations we know nothing about. And we compare ourselves to others without walking in their shoes. We blow things out of proportion, think in absolutes and don't provide concrete evidence.

If you fail a test, you might think that you're a failure. If you make a mistake, you feel like a mistake. In truth, you failed a test. You made a mistake. That's all; feeling these things doesn't make you those things. These acts aren't globally-based. You've done well on other tests. You've done plenty of things correctly in the past. Unfortunately, we often let events overtake us and allow the ensuing emotions to wreak havoc on our sense of well-being. This is a very destructive thought-pattern. It doesn't help anyone.

Throughout our lives, we tell ourselves all kinds of untruths and our brains react emotionally. This is perfectly normal. However, we need to be aware of the captions beneath our thoughts, of the ultra-critical judgment we impose upon ourselves. Almost always, you'll find flaws that should be corrected. Rational thinking is important for everyone and it's absolutely imperative for fetishists. This is because we universally think irrationally. As a result of this, we suffer unnecessarily. We must to learn how to modify our thoughts to reflect the truth instead of skewed, judgmental half-truths.

Most fetishists suffer from anxiety disorder. That's because fetishists are in a constant state of worry. They fear being discovered; they worry about being "caught."

Right now, I want you to do something for me—I want you to focus on your own fetish. Tune into your body and try to define your own feelings about fetish. Are you feeling sad? Angry? Remorseful? Ashamed? Now, I want you to write down what you're telling yourself in the moment. Most fetishists have thoughts that link up to feelings of sadness, anger and embarrassment. They usually sound something like this:

- My life is messed up because I have a fetish.
- If anyone knew what I like, they would lock me up.
- My wife would divorce me if she found out.
- I'm a freak of nature, perverted and sick.

Can you see how your thoughts affect the way you feel? These thoughts would make anyone feel sad, angry and anxious. The thoughts are filled with worry without any real evidence. After all, no one has ever gotten jailed because of a sexual fantasy. You don't know for sure how your wife would react (she might actually like it). And calling yourself names is definitely not helpful. I bet you would never, ever call a friend such cruel names or be so judgmental toward them. Then why treat yourself so harshly?

It's paramount that you work on your own perceptions in order to change the way you feel. If you don't know how to do this, there are tons of psychology books that deal with the subject of Cognitive Behavioral Therapy. Although it's too big of a concept to properly discuss here, the primary premise of this evidence-based theory states that no one has emotion based upon anything outside of themselves. Emotions are produced from our thinking process. And most of the time, this thinking is not based on fact or rationally based.

This is especially true for fetishists. I'll bet that if you examine your thoughts about fetish, they lead you to feel negatively about yourself. For example, if you think:

- My fetish makes me different.
- My fetish is wrong.
- My fetish is abnormal.

Then the above thoughts would produce feelings of shame and guilt. These thoughts are not rational or based on fact.

Instead, a more positive way to think would be:

- My fetish is out of the ordinary, but that's just my fetish.
  My fetish is only one small part of who I am.
- "Wrong" is a very judgmental word. My fetish is
  simply atypical.
- Again, the word "abnormal" is extremely judgmental and
  labeling. My fetish is simply different. After all, who's to
  say what's normal and what's not normal?

When you say the first three statements out loud, I guarantee you will feel depressed and anxious. When you repeat the modified thoughts, I guarantee you will feel grounded and at peace with yourself.

Give Yourself a Break

We think that our fetish is wrong and so we are now wrong. This kind of thinking is dangerous and toxic. But it's the very act of thinking that can turn it around for you.

Here comes my mantra again: fetish is strong, powerful and never goes away. As a result, your fetish is here to stay. You can choose to think badly of yourself, call yourself names and make dire predictions about your future and relationships. Or, you can choose to change your mode of thought. You can decide to welcome your fetish into your life and embrace it as part of you—just like your kind eyes and your warm smile.

If it's true that fetish is a part of you, then you should approach it differently. You must challenge the old ideas. What is the real truth about your fetish? Does it really make you completely different than everyone or just a little different? Aren't there many things about you which make you the same as everyone else? Is your fetish really harmful? Don't you have many desirable qualities with or without your fetish? Take a moment to formulate the real truth about yourself and the many amazing things that make you tick.

Most people believe that they have no control over their thoughts. Indeed, we are conditioned to blame our spouses, our environment or our situations when we feel angry. We naturally look for situational triggers which we use to explain our anger, sadness, pain or happiness.

Here's a life-changing piece of information: We have no control over people, places or things. However, we have 100% control over how we interpret the events and people in our lives. This seems so basic but it's true. We subject ourselves to all sorts of rigid mind games that hinder instead of help our self-image. I outline a handful of them here:

Labeling

When we call ourselves a weirdo, a pervert or a freak, we are stamping ourselves with a negative label. These loaded words are guaranteed to create feelings of sadness, confusion and anger. It's simply not nice to call yourself names, yet you do. Think about it. Do these words really describe you 100%? Aren't you also kind, truthful and hard-working? Can any one word really describe exactly who you are or describe who anyone is? Aren't you being dishonest when you give yourself a label that doesn't really describe you?

It's important to be accurate with your usage of words. Scientifically speaking, our brains interpret language literally. When you call yourself names, the brain just hears the negative word and acts accordingly. That's why we have to be careful of how we think.

A more truthful approach would be the thought, "My fetish doesn't define me." This statement is neutral. It's a plain fact and fosters more neutral types of feelings.

Calling yourself names isn't polite. Would you ever speak so harshly to a loved one? I doubt it. So, how about being kinder to yourself? Choose the words you call yourself as carefully as you choose the words you'd say to a friend. Be nice!

Thinking in Terms of Black or White

When you call yourself names, you're not looking at yourself honestly. All of us are on a spectrum. Yes, our fetish might be somewhat different, quirky or out-of-the-box, however, it's so much more complex than being all bad.

Inflexible, black-and-white thinking patterns lead to feeling depressed and hopeless. "I'm abnormal," you tell yourself. Well, that's certainly a discouraging thought!

When you think about dating, you feel worried and anxious. "No one will want me because of my fetish," you drum into your brain. "I'm destined to be alone the rest of my life." With thoughts like these, who wouldn't want to give up and resign themselves to a life of lonely masturbation!

When you think inflexibly, you blow your fetish way out of proportion and reason from a place of shame. As a result, you probably feel depressed because your thoughts are judgmental and harsh. You feel anxious because you adapt a way of thinking that teaches you that different is wrong. But it's not—it's merely different.

Black-and-white thinking is almost always tied to feelings of depression. When you tell yourself, "I'll never get someone to understand me" or "I'll always be a captive of my fetish," you aren't factoring in gradients. You're not considering shades of gray and variables. More truthfully, it might take more of an effort to get a partner to understand your sexual fantasies. It might mean that you will have to be diligent in your search for a partner but it's an absolute falsehood to tell yourself that you will "never" find a partner or that you will "always" be alone.

Black-and-white thinking goes hand in hand with depression, lethargy and a general sense of hopelessness. Be careful of falling prey to this destructive pattern of thinking.

False Prophetic Thinking

It's very common to make false predictions in our thinking. Thoughts like, "If anyone knew what I fantasize about, they'd commit me" or "I'm doomed to a life of loneliness" are examples of prophetic thinking based on fear rather than fact. The truth is, you have no real evidence of how anyone will react to your sexual fantasy. You have no ability to accurately predict your future.

Prophetic-type thinking is always anxiety-based. In it, you predict doom based upon fears. The fact is that you are not a fortune teller, psychic or prophet. You feel anxious about the fact that you have a fetish. You tell yourself that bad things will befall you because you're different.

Prophetic thinking is particularly dangerous because false prophesies create anxiety. Anxiety requires quick relief. Quick relief often comes in the form of masturbation and correlates with the fetishistic behavior. Do you see where this is going? It's a vicious cycle. Often, people are so anxious that they turn to their fetish for relief only to access even more negative thinking and self hatred.

It's important to catch yourself—and correct yourself—when you find yourself predicting the future. You'll know you're doing this when your thoughts begin with words like "What if…" and "I know I'll never…"

When you find yourself predicting the future, ask yourself if you have any concrete evidence to back yourself up. Since you're talking about the future, you won't be able to show real proof because the future hasn't happened yet. And what you're so convinced of might never become a reality.

Judgmental Thinking

People have an odd way of talking unkindly to ourselves. When we tell ourselves that fetish is wrong, dirty, and crazy, we are thinking rigidly and casting judgment. When we think this way, we really begin to feel badly about ourselves. We're telling ourselves that we're bad or wrong because we have something out of the norm that turns us on. We are being harsh and hypercritical. In fact, we talk to ourselves in a voice that we would never use with anyone else. It's a disparaging voice that has no purpose other than to lower our self-esteem and cause us to hang our heads in shame.

Fetishists can be very unkind with and condemnatory of themselves. When you find yourself thinking this way, catch yourself and change your tone of inner-voice to something more open, caring and nurturing. Be the kind mother, instead of the abusive one. Be a nurturing teacher, instead of the one who scolds. I know you can do it with a bit of practice.

What if You Came to a Different Way of Thinking about Your Fetish?

I have high hopes that you can—and will!—change the way you think about your fetish. Acceptance is key. The concept is basic, easy to understand and absolutely factual. As a fetishist, you simply don't fit into the norm. That's it, pure and simple. You're not a monster and you're not a freak of nature.

Now, that being said, you have two choices:
1. You can choose to feel bad about yourself; or
2. You can choose to embrace your uniqueness.

The choice is entirely up to you. Listen carefully: I said choice. You can choose to think of yourself as an aberration because you have a fetish. You can choose to believe that no one will like you or accept you because you have a fetish. Or you can choose to understand, manage and accept your fetish.

Self-acceptance is the key to feeling better. Change your thinking about fetish and you can change the way you feel about fetish. New, more evolved thinking will eventually help you reach the goal of true self-compassion and inner peace. We need to think differently about fetish. Rational, healthy thinking is the key to radical acceptance and tranquility of mind.

Some Real-Life Examples:

Example # 1 - Bob, a Foot Fetishist:

Bob has a fetish for women's feet—and not just any feet. For Bob, the feet have to be somewhat dirty and a little bit smelly. In addition, he likes the toenails to be longish and painted bright red. The image and ensuing odor is intoxicating to Bob and produce a guaranteed erection. In the past, Bob has been able to bring his fantasy to life with more than one partner. He also likes to masturbate to images of feet which he has personally photographed. When Bob is engaging in his fantasy, he's obviously extremely happy. However, when it's over and he has orgasmed, Bob runs into trouble with himself—he feels depressed, hopeless and embarrassed.

Bob's Thoughts:
- There's something very wrong with me.
- I'll never get better.

Distortions:

Can you see the distortions in Bob's thinking? When Bob says there's something wrong with him, he thinks solely in terms of black and white. He doesn't consider all that is right with him. Instead, he's extremely judgmental and makes future predictions without any real evidence.

Modified Thoughts:
- True, I have a foot fetish but that fetish doesn't define who I am.
- I can learn to embrace my fetish rather than try to change myself.
- I have plenty of good qualities. I just have to learn how to accept myself.

Example # 2 - Johnny, a Panty Fetishist:

Johnny has a fetish for silk. More specifically, bikini panties with strings on the side. He loves to see women clad in string bikinis. He also loves to feel the material against his own skin. Sometimes Johnny indulges in the fetish by wearing the panties himself and masturbating. But Johnny also has issues with his fetish. He wants to be open with his girlfriend about it but he's worried about her reaction.

Johnny's Thoughts:
- I shouldn't be so focused on panties.
- It's especially wrong for me to wear panties as a man. What if someone found out?
- I'll never live a normal life if I continue to indulge in my fetish.

Distortions:

Johnny's thinking is very much based on the future. This produces feelings of anxiety. Whenever you say "what if" anxiety always follows. He also thinks judgmentally about himself and thinks in terms of black and white.

Modified Thoughts:
- I have a panty fetish and it's here to stay.
- I enjoy wearing panties, so what? Other people's thoughts won't harm me.
- I can learn to incorporate this fetish into my life as much or as little as I want. It's all up to me.

Example # 3 – Craig, an Adult Baby

Craig has a diaper fetish and would like to explore infantilism with a willing partner. To date, he indulges in his fetish by sometimes wearing diapers to bed and looking at adult material geared towards infantilism. Once in a blue moon, he takes some time to "baby" himself at home. Craig feels great while he's doing it, but afterwards, feels embarrassed, foolish, lonely and self-conscious.

Craig's Thoughts:
- This fetish means that I'm very sick.
- I would just die if anyone found out what I do.
- I don't deserve the bliss I feel when I engage in my babying activities.

Distortions:
Craig is being judgmental. He's the one who's calling himself names that lead to feeling bad about himself. The truth of the matter is that Craig doesn't know exactly how he would feel if someone found out—he might actually feel relieved. Craig is jumping to conclusions. He's also being disapproving when he says that he doesn't deserve to feel good. Every human being deserves to feel good, even fetishists!

Modified Thoughts:
- I'm unfairly judging the fetish. Having a fetish just means I'm different, not sick.
- I'm being overly dramatic about dying. If I accept my fetish, chances are good that others will accept it, too. And if they

don't accept me, I don't want them in my life.
- Of course, I deserve to feel good. This is only one way that makes me feel good but I enjoy this fetish and it doesn't hurt anyone.

Now It's Your Turn

How about you? What do you tell yourself about your fetish? Write down your thoughts. Can you identify any distortions? If so, write down the distortions and try to explain why they're untruthful. Modify your thoughts so that they're more rational. Now jot down your modified thoughts.

In Summary

It's not the fact that you have a fetish which is the problem. Your problem is the way you think about your fetish. Your negative thoughts lead you to feelings of self-hatred, loathing, anger, severe depression and worry. You've been programmed to talk to yourself in a voice that's self-deprecating, hostile, and narrow-minded. That's because you've internalized the early messages given to you by parents, teachers and a puritanical society. You've bought into the nonsense that just because you deviate from the norm, you're a deviant. Just because your wishes stray from the traditionally romantic norm doesn't mean you're not romantic. This simply is not the case.

Remember that you aren't feeling anxious, guilty or shameful because you have a fetish. You feel this way because of the negatives messages you've internalized and adapted as your own. Make sure you're conscious of your thoughts. Notice the fallacies. Change these untruths to honest observations. When you do this, you're guaranteed to feel better. Adjusting your way of thinking will serve you and ultimately create feelings of inner peace and acceptance.

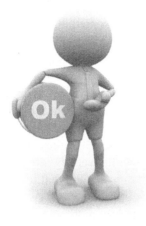

Chapter 6 - The Benefits of Acceptance

Let's recap what we've done in the first five chapters of this book:

- You've educated yourself about what fetish is and isn't.
- You've learned that your negative thinking about your fetish doesn't help you feel the way you'd like to feel about yourself.
- You've examined your thought process about fetish and identified distortions.
- And finally, you've modified your thinking in order to come to a place of self-acceptance.

Now you're at a pivotal point in learning to have control of your fetish.

Congratulations!

What is Acceptance?

Acceptance is the realization that fetish plays only a small role in defining who you are as a human being. Fetish simply means that there is something different or quirky about your arousal triggers. Your proclivities are out-of-the-box but it doesn't mean that you're out-of-the-box. You have made a conscious decision to love yourself as you are. You are no longer conflicted. You are no longer trying to fight it or will it away. You have surrendered to the fact that your fetish is here to stay.

Your self-talk about fetish is rationally based. You no longer put yourself down, call yourself names or make dire predictions about how your fetish will adversely affect your life. You are now well educated and understand that fetish does not dictate how you will spend your life.

Soon we will be focusing more on your fetish and identifying what it entails. We will be defining the details and learning what parts of the fetish are most important to you. We will then be making a rational decision about how you will ultimately choose to incorporate fetish into your life.

But for now, let's talk more about self-understanding and why it's so important. You know who you are. You don't need to be apologetic. You can zero in on who you are and present yourself to the world emphasizing all of your positive attributes. The fact that you have a fetish doesn't have to bring you down. You can embrace it for what it is and actually turn it into something fun and positive. There are many things about your fetish that you can champion. Yes, you can turn lemons into lemonade!

If you take a moment to think about it, there are some pretty cool things about having a fetish, including, but not limited to:

1. You have something that reliably turns you on.

Most long-term married couples complain that sex begins to get a little boring as the years roll by. They say it's the same routine and no matter how much they try. There are only so many ways to perform the same old act. Because of this, many couples search for ideas to spice things up. Sadly, some long-term partners barely want to have erotic relations after years of being together. Their interest in sex often wanes. But this is not true for the fetishist.

Your sex drive is here to stay. Because your fetish drive is so powerful, you will have a solid source to feed feelings of arousal until the day you die. Thinking of your fetish is a guarantee that your penis will work and you'll be ready to go. And since there are many variations within each fetish, if you want to get adventurous, there are plenty of ways to spice things up. You are limited only by your own imagination and creativity. In this way, you are really lucky to have a fetish because it will reliably turn you on for the rest of your life. It's ever-present, ever-ready and here to stay. That's a good thing!

2. Your partner will also be able to remain active with you.

This is something to consider when you think about sharing your fetish with your partner. If she's willing to participate even a little bit, you will have an active sex life way beyond menopause visits her and well into your Golden Years. Even if her own sex drive wanes, your bedroom can still be an active place.

You and your partner will always have a way to carnally connect because fetish is not connected to traditional intercourse alone. Your partner only has to be willing, understanding and have a desire to please. She can rest assured that as long as she joins in with something connected to your fetish, you'll find her sexy and desirable for the rest of her days. She'll always be able to get you going with verbiage, props or performing some kind of act. She'll know what to say and what to do. She'll be aware of your sexual triggers and hotspots.

Women who are married to fetishists don't know how lucky they are. If you and your partner can jump on the Fetish Train, she can rest assured that you'll never stray and she'll always be the star of your sexual fantasies.

3. Fetish doesn't get boring.

Most fetishists are bright people. They have wonderful imaginations and fetish holds many possibilities for them. Though there is a repetitive nature with some fetishes, they can often be expanded upon. There are countless ways to dominate, if that's your thing. There are tons of roles to be played out and many different fetish scenarios to re-enact.

Your sex life can be interesting and exciting as long as you give yourself permission to explore. The more you accept yourself, the more your mind will expand. And if you run out of ideas, the Internet is always available to offer new options. We live in a day and age where there's tons of useful information online. Many, many fetishists are coming out and are happy to share in something that provides true bliss.

4. You're thinking more rationally.

You've thought negatively about your fetish for decades. Since your current thoughts are newer, they must be reinforced. If you ever find yourself feeling down or frustrated about your fetish, remember to take heed of what you're thinking about in the moment. Write down the thought and make sure it's rational. If not, remember to quickly revise the thought so that you will feel back in control.

Be patient with yourself. Your old ideas have been with you all your life. They didn't develop overnight. I know you're loving the idea of acceptance right now, and intellectually it makes sense. But sometimes new ideas take a while to become a part of you. It takes time for you to process and "own" the thought. It's kind of like the difference between reading a book about surfing and actually riding the wave.

Trust me, your new idea of self-acknowledgement can become a definitive part of your makeup. It just takes practice, time and patience.

5. Acceptance leads to well-being and confidence.

When you accept yourself as you are, you will feel confident. You will experience improved self-esteem. Instead of battling something you can't change, you will have the sense of calm necessary for you to focus in on the present things in your life. You'll have time to concentrate on work, your family and enjoying your life in the moment. If you choose to indulge your fetish, you will do so with a spirit of enjoyment. By removing your anxiety level, your fetish time will be scheduled by choice and it won't be about "self-soothing."

Be kind and gentle with yourself. Remember all the good things about you and the accomplishments you're proud of.

Think about the little things you do each day that enhances the lives of others. Sometimes it can be as small as smiling at a stranger or giving some spare change to the homeless. Every human being has worth and value. I know that you realize this as well.

Embrace all that makes you the good person you are. I invite you to enjoy a sense of inner-contentment and self-compassion. Take a little time to experience this tranquility. Savor it. Revel in it. You deserve it.

The next nine chapters will help you to understand and define your fetish. Once you have acquired this knowledge, you will make a rational decision about how you want to incorporate fetish into your life. You'll decide if you want to share it with your present or future partner, a paid professional or if you just want to keep it to yourself.

But no matter what you choose, it's important to think about all the details of your fetish. This is good information for you to have and it's absolutely necessary if you want to share your fetish with another person.

For now, I invite you to take pleasure in your feeling of self-acceptance and move onto your own path of self-exploration when you feel you're ready to forge ahead. I'll be there when you are.

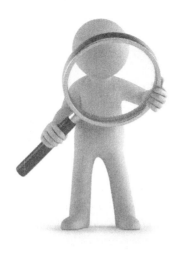

Chapter 7 - Identification

Identification requires you to hone in on and define your fetish needs. It's not enough merely to label your fetish. You must take an honest inventory in order for you to understand all of its fine nuances. You must know whether or not your fetish is straightforward or more complex. You should establish whether your fetish is multifaceted with a variety of components. You have to figure out exactly what your fetish entails so that you can make thoughtful choices about how to best incorporate fetish into your life.

Once you take the time to identify what your fetish does and does not entail, it will enable you to communicate your desires to another human being if you so choose. It will also help you to know what aspects of fetish fulfillment are necessary as opposed to optional. The choice is all in your hands.

You have to understand all aspects of your fetish to truly know if there's any room for compromise or variety. For example, you might fantasize about being dominated and kissing a female foot. But you have to establish which need is essential. Domination? Foot worship? Or does it have to be both?

Another example of compromise or variety is that you might fantasize about rubber and latex. But is it critical for you and your partner to both wear the material or can you make a concession with just her (not you) donning a pair of rubber or latex boots?

And finally, here's one more example. You might like the idea of giving and receiving spankings, but could you compromise with allowing your "vanilla" partner to give you spankings since she might not like the idea of receiving pain? (By the way, "vanilla" is a term that refers to something that involves no kink or twists.)

Identification will also be important if you choose to see a professional sex worker for fetish fulfillment. The more she knows, the better your session will be. Identification will ensure that you are aware of your points of arousal, attitude, roles and variables that make the fetish uniquely yours. No two fetishists are exactly alike. Now's the time to figure out what makes the fetish belong to you, what makes it personal.

Some fetishes are very straightforward, meaning that there's an object, body part or act that arouses the fetishist. Most people wouldn't associate these things with sexual arousal, but you do. This is your fetish and now you're ready to own it. Being urinated on, kissing a boot, dressing like a plush animal, seeing a woman's lips painted glossy red, a woman blowing smoke in your face… These turn-ons are uniquely yours. Only you can define what gets you going.

Other fetishes are more complex and have variables that require strategic attention. It's not only about you wearing lingerie but a big component is that you have to feel like you have no choice in doing so. You like the fantasy of your woman being with another man but only if you are thoroughly humiliated. You like to wear diapers but you don't want to be asked to soil them. You like to see women dressed in silk panties but they have to be high-cut string bikinis as opposed to traditionally-shaped panties. Again, only you can describe your fetish. Only you can identify your turn-ons and cravings. Now that you have self-acceptance, you can stop judging and start investigating.

Below you will find the identified variables to help get you started. These variables can be applied to any fetish. This is your basic checklist. Feel free to add or subtract according to what is important to you.

Chapters 8-15 guide you through the Identification Process. I've dedicated chapters to specific fetishes which are fairly common. This means that I've seen them often through my many years of practice and have personally worked with people who have these fetishes. These chapters illustrate how detailed each fetish can be.

If your particular fetish doesn't appear here, please accept my apology. As I've said, fetishes are as individual as fingerprints and it's impossible to describe them all within the confines of a book. Simply choose a chapter that most closely relates to your fetish and use the example as a guideline. But to make things easier for you, I'm also providing general identification questions in this chapter as well, which can be applied to practically any fetish, no matter how obscure.

I encourage you to adapt any questions that pertain to you. Feel free to add some of your own. I want you to be as thorough as possible. Every detail counts. It might be helpful if you imagine that you're speaking to someone. That someone is a person who offers unconditional positive feedback and is completely nonjudgmental. That person might even be you. The basic idea is to uncover and explain your fetish in intimate detail to a caring human being.

I suggest you write the responses to your Fetish Checklist on a sheet of paper or type them into your computer. Writing down your answers will help with your thought process and make the exercise more effective. Be sure only you have access to your written thoughts and keep the paper in a safe place. Password protection is advisable if you're creating a document on your computer.

FETISH CHECKLIST

Name Your Fetish

Remember that it's not enough to provide a generic label. Please be very specific. Do a little research about your fetish online. By looking it up, your thought process will be sparked and your memory will be jogged.

Talk about how your fetish evolved.
- When exactly did you first discover that you had a fetish.
- Where were you?
- How old were you?
- When did you first act upon the fetish?
- What was the experience like?

Did you have a latency period? Most fetishists have very early memories of their fetish, usually between the ages of six or eight. Then they forget about their fetish until adolescence strikes. However, once they hit puberty, the fetish re-emerges.
- Did your fetish disappear during a latency period?
- Did it re-emerge during puberty?
- Do you remember how you handled your thoughts?
- Were you confused, ashamed or just aroused?
- How did you act upon your fetish when you
  were young?

Specifics
Many people's fetishes are ultra-specific and involve sensory aspects like color, texture, taste and smell. Look deeply into the particulars of your fetish for a moment.
What about your fetish turns you on?
(Be as detailed as possible.)
- What do you think about at the moment of orgasm?
- What drives you over the edge?

What Makes Your Fetish Uniquely Yours?
Remember that there are many variables in each fetish. Think of how your fetish is the same as the information you see online. Ask yourself how is it different? I've listed some prompts below to help you in this process. Think of them as Your Five Fetish Senses.

Your Five Fetish Senses:

Eyes - What image or images do you like to see? Bookmark favorite photos you've seen online. What is it about these images that turns you on? Is it a facial expression? An act? A costume?

Ears - What do you like to hear? Verbiage is extremely important in a fetish, so important that it will get a category of its own. But perhaps there are other sounds that get you going-like the swish of the whip, the crunch of snail being stepped on or the sound of a woman passing gas. List yours.

Nose - What do you like to smell? Perfume? Leather? Latex? Some fetishes require scent. Sense memories are a powerful aphrodisiac. Is there a perfume, oil or food fragrance that does it for you? An unwashed body part? Or maybe a section of the anatomy that needs to be scrubbed with a small amount of soap? Think about the aroma that's required by you.

Mouth - What do you like to taste? Do you enjoy licking a woman's leather? Eating your ejaculation? Tasting the salt from her skin? Take a moment to think and then take note.

Fingertips - What do you like to touch? Are there particular sensations you enjoy giving or receiving? Is there the feel of certain materials that you crave, be it soft, rough, silky or furry?

Costuming

You probably think about this obsessively when you visualize your fetish image. However, if your image requires a particular costume, article of clothing or prop, remember to include it here.

- Be specific! Don't just say high-heeled shoes, write down exactly how high. How many inches? What shape should the heels be? What's the color and material of the shoe?

- Write down every detail of the costume. If it's a skirt, remember to include the length of the skirt, the color and how you'd like it to fit her (tight or loose).

Costuming is an important part of your fetish, so remember to really think hard about what you like. If it's not important, then remember to mention this on your identification list, as well.

Verbiage

Although you probably thought a bit about this during your inventory of Your Five Fetish Senses, words often play an integral part of fantasy fulfillment. Think about the phrases that turn you on. Write them down. Also consider:

- How do you like to hear the words spoken? Loud? Soft? In a harsh voice? An authoritative voice? Shouted or whispered?
- Do you like to hear short commands or details about what you're required to do.
- What voice do you use in the fantasy? Perhaps you're the one in control.
- What voice do you use that makes you feel best?
- What voice would your partner respond to well?
- What kind of "tone" should she have? Bitchy? Submissive? Or sweet?

Remember, voice tone can make or break a scene. Again, be thoughtful about what works best for you. It's all about you here!

Texture

For many, texture plays a starring role in their fetish. How about you?
- Do you prefer rough skin or smooth?
- Soft clothing or coarse?
- Supple or thick material?

After you identify the kind of textures you enjoy, think about the way you like to be handled.
- Roughly or gently?
- Jerked around or softly guided?

Be specific so that you can communicate exactly what you prefer.

Role

This establishes what your partner must do in order to enhance your fetish experience.
- Is she an observer, a passive participant or dominator?
- Does she have to wear a particular garment or costume?
- Should she talk in a certain way? Use particular words?
- Does she have to force you or assist you in fulfilling your fetish?

Attitude

Most of you will agree that attitude is really important fetish-wise. First and foremost, you want to know that she's into your fetish and is having fun. Even if the fetish is not as charged for her as it is for you, you still want to know she's having a good time. Even if it's just the fact that she's enjoying herself because she likes giving pleasure to you.

Within the context of the fetish, attitude is often important as well.
- Should she behave playfully? Seductively? Sadistically?
- Should she take a passive or aggressive stance?

You've done a wonderful job of identifying the basics of your fetish. Now it's time to dig deeper and consider the more complex aspects of your fetish.

Humiliation

Many fetishes involve the aspect of humiliation. How about yours?
- Do you like to play up the aspect of humiliation when acting out your fetish?

You might like to explore your inner feelings of embarrassment or of feeling silly in your fetish. Believe it or not, playing out this emotion is actually very therapeutic. We all feel a little silly at times. Acknowledging and exaggerating inner shame is often a first step toward healing. Exposure or flooding fosters desensitization.

But remember, humiliation must always be done in a spirit of caring and of non-judgment. For example, if you're already sensitive about being overweight, it's no fun to be called fat. However, if you feel a bit ridiculous about being spanked as an adult, you might find it arousing to be called on it. Likewise, if you have an unreasonable obsession about your average-sized penis being too small, a touch of joking might point out the absurdity of your fears.

It's very, very important for you to figure out if the idea of humiliation is part of your scene. You need to determine how it comes into play and what would be comfortable or provide excitement for you. Or not. It's important to realize that the aspect of humiliation isn't part of everyone's fetish. And it doesn't have to be part of yours. Some fetishists enjoy humiliation. Others do not. It's up to you to decide.

So, figure out if there are any deal-breakers that would ruin a scene for you. If there are any words or name-calling that would personally hurt you, make note of them. It's important to have your partner avoid saying them in order for your fetish re-enactment to go as planned. Often, what's not said, is as important as the words you love to hear.

Forced Fetish

This is another point to include in your Identification Process inventory. Many fetishes include an element of force. By being forced, I mean that within your fantasy, you imagine that you're out of control of the situation. You have no choice but to perform an act, wear a piece of clothing or behave in a way that ordinarily you wouldn't.

Now, of course, we know that you want to be doing this act because it's your fetish. But in the realm of some people's fetish, being forced is a very important aspect of it. Only you can decide if it's part of your fantasy or not. And it usually goes one way or the other—there's no middle ground when it comes to being forced.

If being forced is part of your fantasy:
- Do you imagine being forced into wearing diapers as a humiliating punishment?
- Do you prefer to be forced into female clothing for another's enjoyment? (This is a totally different beast than cross-dressing.)
- Do you have the like to be forced to suck on her toes, kiss her buttocks or drink her urine?

It's essential that you seriously consider and write down your responses if being "forced" is a part of your own personal fantasy world.

Turn-Offs

In many ways, turn-offs are as important as turn-ons. So, it's not only key to identify what turns you on but it's equally as important to know what turns you off or what might be upsetting to you. You've got to ask yourself:
- Is there anything that would make you want to stop a scene?
- Is there any act that is abhorrent to you?
- What other things would turn you off? A nervous laugh? A particular word or phrase? Incompetence? Aggressiveness? Mean-spiritedness? Ineptitude?

Identify any mood-killers you anticipate so you can correct them before they begin.

Limits

Many fetishists would consider "turn-offs" as limits. Limits are things that you really don't want to do, a line you really don't want to cross. Please realize that the notion of personal limits has nothing to do with being forced; it's more closely something that horrifies you.

If you're submissive, it's particularly important to know your limits. Many subs will visit a Dominatrix and say that they want to be pushed past their limits and this might be true, but only up to a certain point. Everyone has barriers they don't want to cross, even in fetish or fantasy.

As a therapist, I've noticed clients voicing a distinct area of limits when it comes to the realm of bathroom functions (golden or brown showers, when a person enjoys being urinated upon or shat upon), homosexual acts or acts that are particularly excruciating. These fetishists often relay unpleasant experiences when interacting with a dominant who doesn't ask about, or respect their limits. This is another reason why this Identification Process is so important.

Pain thresholds are different for everyone. Some people can take a horrific spanking on their buttocks area but dislike even the mildest flogger on their backs. Others enjoy having their nipples squeezed but hate any kind of attention paid to their testicles.

In your Identification Process, write down your limits. It's important to know them and be committed to them so that you understand yourself and can clearly communicate your limits to another person.

A Word about Patience

Even after jotting down your fetish "do's and don'ts," no matter how much you communicate, no one is perfect. No one will get your fetish scene exactly right on the first try. It's virtually impossible. Because of this, you might have to lower your expectations, at least in the beginning.

Try your best to enjoy what your partner is willing to do. Appreciation goes a long way. Compliment rather than criticize. Don't be demanding while the scene is going on. Before you even begin, you have to establish a way to communicate how not to stop the scene, just change the action if it becomes too intense. I've gone into this in a bit more detail in the "Safe Words" section that follows.

Most importantly, try to keep your spirits high and continue to completion. Later on, you can give good, constructive feedback. But remember, she's trying her best. Give her the benefit of the doubt.

Safe Words

Again, practice makes perfect. If you're playing with an inexperienced partner, she will make mistakes. That's why safe words are a must. Safe words offer a way the two of you can communicate while the scene is taking place without breaking the mood.

Many use the word "mercy" to stop a scene dead in its tracks. Others use the colors of traffic lights: green for good, yellow to slow down or red to stop completely. You might want to think of words or gestures that would be more personal and more suited to the two of you. But also keep in mind how you can communicate in a way that won't take you out of your aroused state.

In Summary

You are the one and only expert about your personal fetish. The more thoughtful you are, the more you'll be able to make important decisions about how to incorporate fetish into your life.

Use the Fetish Checklist as a general guide to help you identify and then communicate your requirements to a potential partner. This checklist was designed to help you figure out what you like, no matter what your fetish might be.

The following eight chapters will focus on individual fetishes. Because fetishes are complex and unique, they require you to be very specific and thorough when you communicate to your partner.

For each chapter, I chose fetishes that have variables in order to help you formulate your thoughts. I also mention fetishes which are more common and straightforward. Chapter 15, the last one in this section, includes some of the less-common fetishes.

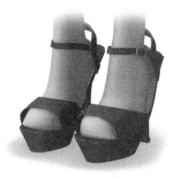

Chapter 8 - Do You Have A Foot Fetish?

If you have a foot fetish, it means you get aroused by looking at, touching or playing with female feet. In fact, you like feet, the way that most men like the buttocks or breasts. In life, we tend to assume that guys are either "tit men" or "ass men," but that's not necessarily the case. This is why "assume" is the perfect word here. There are billions of men in the world, so why do we assume that there are only two sexual triggers on the planet? This means there are potentially billions of sexual triggers out there. All men are not alike. And, as it turns out, a large number of men happen to have a thing for feet. That's just the way it is. You don't have to feel alone because you aren't.

As part of your Identification Process, it's important to be specific about your foot fetish. Although this fetish appears simple on the surface, it can also be extremely complex. It's not enough to say that you have a foot fetish; it's important to know what your fetish actually entails. You might like a woman's feet to touch, caress or massage. You might also like the idea of her using her feet, rather than her hands, to masturbate you to orgasm. You might just like to smell them or you might just want to look at them.

You might like all kinds of feet, generally speaking, but then crave a little something extra. That something extra might be smooth, pedicured toenails painted pink or raggedy feet that are smelly and unwashed. I know one fetishist who likes the soles of the feet to be rough like sandpaper. Within the context of a foot fetish there are many possibilities; they're almost endless.

Many people say they have a foot fetish when in reality they have a fetish for feet encased in shoes or boots. They might also say that they have a fetish for feet when in reality they love a pair of shapely legs. Finally, many foot fetishists enjoy feet within the context of an activity like trampling, toe-sucking or crushing.

In addition to enjoying the look, feel or interaction with the female foot, the "foot man" might also like the idea of Dominant/submissive (D/s) interaction. If that describes you, then you might have what is known as a dual fetish. Meaning, you like foot worship within the context of D/s exchange. The mindset of your fetish then becomes something a little more complex than being a foot fetishist alone. You would then need to identify yourself as a submissive male who's into foot fetish. See how complex it can get?

Foot fetishes appear simple on the surface, yet there could be many facets to them. The Identification Phase will give you the opportunity to understand what your fetish is all about. The more you know, the better you'll be able to communicate your passions to another person. You will also be able to make a rational decision about whether or not your fetish is something that your partner would be able or willing to share with you.

My hope is that you will be identify and then be flexible about your fetish. For example, if you like rough feet, can you compromise with your woman's feet which happen to be naturally soft? If your wife can be persuaded to do some foot play can you be satisfied with that activity and leave the D/s role-play aside?

This is why the Identification Phase is vital to help you make decisions about your fetish. In it, you evaluate your fetish as a whole until you can identify the components and then make some conscious decisions about how to rationally incorporate fetish into your life.

During the Identification Phase, I want you to get in touch with what your fetish is all about. This will help you to understand yourself as well as prepare you to communicate with another person, if you decide to do so.

These questions will help guide you:
- Are you a purist when it comes to feet?
- If you are a true-blue foot fetishist, you simply like female feet. What's your ideal foot image? Small, medium or large?
- Long, medium or short toenails?
- Are the nails round or square?
- Toenail polish or no polish?
- If you like polish, be specific if you have a preference for shade. Many fetishists love fire-engine red or midnight black.
- Are the toes painted one color or do you prefer the new look of multi-colored polish?
- Do you like designs, rhinestones or straight-up polish?
- Are toe rings or ornaments part involved? If so, any particular size, shape or color?
- Do you have a thing for smelly feet?

The list can go on and on. But I think you get the idea. Most women would assume that if they're dating a foot fetishist, they'd better invest in a pedicure. But unbeknownst to them, you might be a fetishist that doesn't like that look. You might prefer coarse soles, no polish and pungent feet. Some foot fetishists love aroma of an unwashed foot. And so on. Do you see where this is going? It's your job to know what you like so you can communicate it to someone else later.

Next, I'll go into some of the things I touched upon earlier in a bit more detail to further pinpoint your self-discovery:

Bare or shod feet?

Again, it would be assumed that a foot fetishist has a fondness for bare feet. This assumption would make sense because men commonly talk about the female anatomy in its naked form. But just like men traditionally like lingerie, your form of lingerie might be what encases her feet, be it stockings, pantyhose or bulky gym socks.

What kind of shoes?

If you like high heels, figure out your heel preference. Short, sensible, matronly pumps or high heels? If you like high heels, then how many inches should they be? Stiletto or spike heels or thick, wedgy platforms? Open or closed-toe shoes? Or you might actually prefer flats, squeaky, white nurse's shoes. I know of fetishists who like sandals, sneakers or even house slippers. Only you have the ability to figure out precisely what you prefer so you can hopefully be able to share with a partner.

Do you like boots?

Some fetishists are turned on by the feet encased in boots. If this is your preference, is your dream boot thigh-high, mid-length or calf-length? Are they leather, latex or rubber rain boots? Sexy boots or no-nonsense Totes? High-heeled boots or flats?

What do you like to do with feet?

Many foot fetishists naturally utilize the foot during foreplay. If you simply enjoy massaging, touching or licking toes, you might be able to naturally incorporate these activities into your sexual repertoire. Especially if you don't require any particular look or foot adornment.

Footplay as Foreplay

It isn't difficult to casually interact with your woman's feet during lovemaking. Admittedly, it's kind of a sneaky way of getting your needs met—without even having to share your fetish. That's something you have to figure out for yourself, how comfortable you are with this type of interaction. However, it is a viable option if you're simply a guy who loves to interact with feet.

One way to work footplay into your erotic repertoire is to start with a brief foot massage. Who doesn't like a foot massage? Some men think giving a foot massage is just as carnal as penetrative sex. Remember Jules and Vincent's discussion in *Pulp Fiction*?

So, first see if she's receptive to being touched on that part of her body. Be cognizant of any hyper-sensitivity. Many people are really ticklish on the bottom of their feet. This doesn't mean you have to stop, but you might have to readjust your touch. Generally speaking, a firmer touch is less stimulating or less ticklish than a soft caress with just your fingertips. Watch her reaction. Always be respectful of what is pleasing or not pleasing to her.

If you do indeed enjoy sucking on her toes or even putting her whole foot into your mouth, approach slowly and with caution. If you move gradually lovingly and confidently, chances are that you will get what you want. But don't just dive in. A little bit at a time. Treat her as carefully as you would a virgin, because in many respects, she is.

What verbiage or attitude do you require?

A pure foot fetishist is only interested in the feet. Period. Therefore, you wouldn't need your woman to say anything or assume any kind of role. Feet are your focus and your favorite part of her anatomy.

As I discussed earlier, you might like bare feet, smelly feet or feet encased in treacherously-high heels, strappy scandals or chunky boots. Whatever the case, all you require is a willing partner who has an open mind and wants to play.

The only communication lies within your personal esthetics and particular "likes." You can tell her to come to bed barefoot or to wear shoes. You can ask her to present you with tootsies that are scrupulously clean or downright dirty. Manicured or natural, unvarnished toenails. After that, it's pretty simple. All she has to do is lie back, relax and enjoy the sensations you create. The fetish play is very much in your control.

Domination Vs. Foot Fetish

Foot fetishists often like to worship feet within the context of Dominant/submissive relationships. If that's you, it's important to figure out exactly what you like so you can communicate correctly to your partner. Or you might decide that you don't want to tell this to your partner at all. That's fine, too. You just have to weigh out which is more important—foot play or domination? The Identification Process discussed in the previous chapter will give you the answers you seek.

Are you a submissive male who likes feet?

If you feel you're submissive, then your foot fetish is linked with female domination. Translation: You prefer to enact your fetish when you're in a subservient position. In fact, you might not be into feet unless you're engaged in a Dominant/submissive scene. In this case, you probably wouldn't be content to incorporate foot worship into traditional lovemaking. That just wouldn't cut it for you.

Instead, you might be someone who's more interested in playing out Dominant/submissive role-play fantasies. Foot, heel or boot worship is generally part of the scene but the worship aspect takes second place to being ordered or forced to engage with a woman's feet. For you, worshiping the foot falls within the context of being given specific orders. You like the idea that a Dominant female is providing direction. And you like taking her directions when they specifically involve lavishing love and affection upon her feet.

Some submissive foot fetishists crave being told to get on their knees and administer light kisses all over the foot or on specific parts of the feet or legs. Other fetishists enjoy licking each toe separately or taking the whole foot in the mouth in a way that mimics penetrative intercourse. Some fetishists want to kiss the top of the shoes and others want to lick the soles of the boot or shoes...the dirtier the better. Figure out your own triggers and hot spots.

Are you a submissive male who has a forced foot fetish?

When foot worship is incorporated into a D/s scene, some fetishists like the idea of being forced. This is very different than merely being "ordered' or told what to do. The mindset here drifts into the area of humiliation. In your fantasy, you think the idea of foot worship is degrading, dirty and embarrassing. Your Dominant partner is requiring this act of contrition in order to put you in your place. She wants you to feel lowly, therefore she roughly shoves her foot or boot into your mouth, sometimes to the point that you are gagging. (Sometimes the very act of gagging on a foot is part of the turn-on.)

The "forced" mindset allows you to do what you want to do anyway. However, within the context of forced foot fetish, you have "no choice" but to obey. It's different than the submissive who worships to be pleasing. If you like to be forced, you enjoy the idea of losing control. If being forced is your bag, ask yourself these questions:

- What verbiage do you like to hear?
- Do you want to be physically forced, gestured to or told to get into position?
- How do you want to be ordered to tend to your partner's feet?
- What tone of voice should your partner use to communicate with you? A harsh tone, an angry tone or just a very, very assertive tone?
- What are your turn-offs when it comes to your foot fetish?

As much as something turns us on, the same thing can also turn us off if it goes too far. With that in mind, ask yourself:

- Is anything that can ever be said or done to you that would push your limits?
- Is there anything foot-related that would cross your personal boundaries?
- What don't you like about the female foot?
- Is there any act associated with sex and feet that you wouldn't like? (And don't tell me that you like it all because there's a good chance you wouldn't want her foot up your behind! Or would you?)

In Summary

Only you can figure out the components that make up your own fetish. Be thoughtful and take your time. Like any fetish or activity, you might discover new things down the road. When you're comfortable and wish to explore, your mind might even open to new possibilities. You might want to incorporate some toe-sucking into your foot massage. Or, you might like the idea of being forced to do the activities you that initially found frightening. Turn your fear into excitement and figure out exactly what you want. Then go do it.

And most importantly, be honest, thoughtful and courageous in your Identification Process. You'll be so glad you did because it can only bring you closer to achieving your desires.

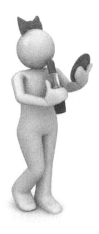

Chapter 9 - Are You A Cross-Dresser?

If you enjoy the idea of donning female garments, your fetish is known as cross-dressing. You've probably been into this fetish ever since you can remember.

For some of you, this fetish may have been "born" way before you can remember. It might be that you had a mother who wanted a daughter rather than a son and dressed you in girls' clothes for her own amusement. Or you could have had sisters who enjoyed teasing you by putting you in their outfits. These family members might have dressed you in "girly" clothes when you were so young, you have no memory of it.

Alternately, you yourself may have raided your sister's closet and tried on her clothes out of curiosity. I know of one man who remembered taking his cousin's panties from the clothes dryer for the purpose of masturbation. The early pleasure from the sensation of the panties on his skin turned into a full-blown fetish when puberty hit and he became sexual. If you think back, you might be able to pinpoint how your own fetish began. Or it could be something that you simply enjoy without rhyme or reason. All you know is that you like some form of cross-dressing.

Cross-dressing is a fetish that exists on a wide spectrum. You can dress a little or a lot. On one end of this spectra are those who merely enjoy wearing one feminine article of clothing, like panties, for example. On the other end of the spectra are those who go for the total transformation. This means that they wear full female attire from head to foot including hair, makeup, underclothes, shoes and accessories.

As for yourself, you might dress alone or secretly wear panties or stockings under your jeans. Or you might like to dress up in full female regalia when you're home alone. Some of you are content to keep this a solo activity but many of you long to share this with your partner and hit the mall together like girlfriends.

Female attire may be your passion. You love to learn as much as you can about styles, makeup and fashion. You're the guy who has a secret closet fit for a princess—and you're the princess. Your impressive collection fulfills every possible mood, fantasy and womanly impulse. You've carefully arranged clothes for work, a night out on the town and luxury lingerie (just in case). You have stacks of wigs, piles of makeup and jewelry to go with every outfit. You can't wait for the opportunities to dress. Dressing makes you feel amazing and beautiful.

However, as good as dressing like a woman makes you feel, it also makes you feel awful about yourself. You're the guy who purges his entire collection of female finery every six months to a year. Even though it kills you, still, you throw it all away. But eventually, your desire to dress overtakes your desire to fit into the public's norms. So you restock, dress again, but the cycle continues. Purge, shop, dress. Purge, shop, dress.

There's also a midpoint on the cross-dressing spectrum. Middle-of-the-roaders are the fellows who dress a little every now and again. You might occasionally like to wear lingerie and don a skirt or dress, but that's about it. No hair or makeup. Your desire to dress comes and goes. You too might purge but since you don't own so many clothes to begin with, throwing things away is not as traumatic as the cross-dresser with a walk-in closet full of attire.

Why do you dress?

Here, I'll be asking you to think about what you like about cross-dressing. Some of you are simply curious. Others crave the thrill of the forbidden. But many of you just enjoy the sensation of the soft fabrics against your skin. It's really a tactile need.

One man I've encountered has a thing for lacy tutus or crinolines. When he donned his ballerina skirt, he felt hypersexual and could stay erect for hours. There was only one problem with his "Crinoline Viagra:" the outfit was a turn off for the ladies. The rejection became unbearable for him. I met this man when he gave up on his fetish and vowed to become celibate. I begged to differ and convinced him otherwise. My plan has given new life to his tutu and his sex life. He was able to find an open-minded lady who realized that sex with a crinoline was pretty great with an avid lover. The fact that Joel is also an extremely intelligent, successful man who treats her well also contributed to her acceptance.

However, regardless of the fact of whether or not a partner embraced his fetish or not, Joel's always been a wonderful guy who happened to have a fetish. Now that he's accepted himself, dealt with his shame and learned how to present his fetish in a positive way, it's made all the difference in Joel's social life. My belief is that this can happen to you, too. You just have to follow the plan I've laid out for you here.

Reasons for cross-dressing are as different as the reasons you might like certain foods. Some of you enjoy cross-dressing for purposes of embarrassment. How many of you were teased by girls when you were young? Even though the name-calling felt shameful, the female attention still felt arousing. Somewhere along the way you began to associate humiliation with being aroused. Hence, your yen for dressing like a girl.

It's time for you to identify what cross dressing means to you, and I'm right here to help guide you. Are you a cross-dresser for the sensuality of the fabric? Or is your impetus because you enjoy seeing yourself as a member of the opposite sex? Is cross dressing representative of being forced or dominated? Only you can articulate what cross dressing means to you.

Here's a list of questions to help you pinpoint your inclination more clearly:

When did you first realize that you were a cross-dresser?

Your early memories are important. They are key in helping you understand your fetish and your needs. Being teased by your sisters might account for your subsequent wish to be humiliated. If you snuck clothing out of the closet and dressed alone, that would explain your preference to dress alone.

Is cross-dressing a sexual turn-on?

You might be driven by the idea of transformation. It's exciting to think of yourself as a female. You dress up and imagine what it feels like to be made love to as a woman. It's almost like understanding sex from the opposite vantage point. Think about how this does or doesn't apply to you.

Some cross-dressers report that dressing isn't as much of a turn-on as it is soothing. Many fetishes are used to quell anxiety. People distract themselves with fantasy play in much the same way as watching sports, going to the gym or escaping into a captivating book. While most fetishes are closely linked to sexual arousal, cross-dressing is sometimes linked to producing good feelings. Often, these good feelings then lead to feeling sexual, which is a different kind of good. When these erotic feelings are produced, that's when you'll be inclined to masturbate in your outfit.

What do you think about at the moment of orgasm?

While masturbating, what are you thinking about? Are you imagining yourself as a woman? A woman home alone pleasuring herself? Or are you thinking about being ravished by your lover? Is your lover a male or a female?

I know that some of you might have "heterosexual" fantasies while being a girl and then worry that you are secretly gay. Don't be concerned—this doesn't mean that you are gay. Most cross-dressers are perfectly straight. However, they have fantasies about being with a man because they really want to know sex from the female point of view. Please don't worry.

The same is true if you imagine being sexual with a woman while dressed as a woman—which is the same as being a woman, in your mind. Who isn't turned on by a little lesbian activity? You also happen to love women and can't even fathom being with anyone but a woman. So, relax, and enjoy your fantasies.

Do you like being penetrated while dressed?

If you are aroused by the idea of anal play, butt plugs or dildos, you probably also have a "strap-on fetish." Again, this doesn't mean you're gay. Instead, you are actually extremely sexually evolved since you have the ability to imagine yourself in another role, as another body. This is rooted in curiosity, not in homosexuality. Since women are penetrated during sex, you want to have a real, authentic experience. So what? It's a fantasy, and fantasies are harmless.

These days it's becoming more and more acceptable for men to admit that they enjoy some kind of dildo and strap-on play. There are physiological reasons for this—it actually feels great to have your prostrate stimulated. And the kinky image of your woman strapping on a dildo is both fascinating and exciting for you personally. It's completely okay to have this fantasy or to indulge in dildo play by yourself. It feels good and the anus is definitely an erogenous zone.

FYI, these days lots of women love the idea of a little role reversal. It gives them the opportunity to know what it feels like to have a penis. The fact that your lady can penetrate you while you're dressed up could add an exciting twist. For the right partner.

Do you dress because you like the texture of the material?

Many men like to dress simply for the tactile aspect. They like to experience the sensations offered by specific articles of clothing. If this sounds like you, what's your favorite material? Silk, satin or soft, sensual cotton?

Is your cross-dressing just about wearing panties?

Many men just want to wear panties. It's as cut and dry as that. They love the feel of creamy silk or satin against their bare skin. They love the way the garments hug their penis and testicles. This may be all you like and that's fine. There is no right or wrong way to be a cross-dresser. It's simply based upon what you enjoy doing.

Just to clarify, panties don't have to be the sole female garment you like. I know of some who have a penchant for pantyhose, bras or even angora sweaters. (Remember the movie *Ed Wood* and his love of angora?) Others like old-fashioned corsets or girdles.

This is your Identification Process, so please be specific about what you like to wear.

Do you like to cross-dress fully?

You might be more into total transformation. This would mean that you enjoy being a female from head to toe. You'd be wearing panties, a bra, stockings, a garter belt, shoes and an exquisite outfit, all painstakingly selected. Hair and makeup is part of your complete package.

So, what does the transformation mean to you? Is it about the image? The art? Or the genuine curiosity about being a girl?

Do you like "Petticoat Punishment"?

Petticoat Punishment actually dates back to the Victorian Era. It was used as a form of discipline to humiliate an errant male—making him wear a woman's petticoat to "teach him a lesson." However, you might enjoy enacting these kinds of role-plays.

Not only would you fantasize about being forced to wear a frilly crinoline slip but you might also imagine (and crave!) being called things like "sissy," "pantywaist" or "brat." Verbiage is important for you to identify because the names you imagine are specific to your fantasy.

Hand in hand with Petticoat Punishment come props such as carrying a purse or a doll.

You might also seek public humiliation to complete your perfect cross-dressing picture.

What kind of cross-dressing image are you going for?

There are all kinds of ways to cross-dress and you probably have your own specific tastes. Do you like to look prim or proper? Loose or slutty? Like a fairy princess? An office girl?

A squeaky-clean nurse in gum-soled shoes? An Army brat with plenty of attitude? Maybe all of the above, depending on your mood.

Does your female image impact your own feelings about women? Or are you merely creating a fantasy story that is very different from your own life. What a wonderful way to escape!

Is your cross-dressing fetish about being "forced"?

The notion of being coerced into dressing up is a super-important variable. You might like the idea of being forced to cross-dress for a woman's sadistic pleasure. The idea of being forced takes the responsibility off your shoulders. Remember that old saying "The Devil made me do it?" It's kind of like that. You relinquish all responsibility when you're made to do something.

In your head, you don't want to dress but you have no choice. This is a very ingenious way of getting yourself off the hook, so to speak. It's a very effective way of perhaps dealing with your own shame. It helps you deal with your inner conflicts concerning cross-dressing.

Please don't over analyze your desires if being forced comes into play with your cross-dressing. This is just part of your fantasy. And remember your mantra—fetish is strong, powerful and doesn't go away. If being forced is part of your cross-dressing menu, it's simply an integral part of your cross-dressing experience. That's it. No self-judgment required.

For purposes of your Identification Process, think about your fantasy. Who is forcing you? What is she like? Is she a Dominatrix, a woman in power like a member of the military, for example, or simply a strict femme fatale like an irresistible Mata Hari? Are you being forced for purposes of punishment or humiliation? Do you enjoy being laughed at or ridiculed?

What kind of verbiage do you like to hear?

While being dressed, what kinds of words complete the picture? Again, if you like to be forced, the verbiage will lean more toward embarrassment rather than about what a pretty girl you are. You might like to be called a "sissy" or a "pantywaist."

If there's an overtly sexual edge to your dressing, words like "whore" or "slut" might fit your personal script better.

But whatever it is, think about the words that enhance your cross-dressing experience. Verbiage is an essential ingredient of the Identification Process.

Do you have a name for your alter ego?

Okay, time to fess up! Do you have a pet name for yourself when you're dressed? If so, what's your female name? Is it something feminine like Lydia, something old-fashioned like Mildred or something sexually-ambiguous like Pat?

If you haven't had the nerve to give yourself a name but are dying to, now's the time to christen your alter ego. Don't be bashful.

What do you want to do when you're dressed?

If you become aroused when you're cross-dressing, then it's off to the bedroom for you. There's no mystery about that one! Often, the fabric or garment alone is so stimulating that you'll climax within moments.

Or you might prefer being a woman in another sense. You want to savor the female experience. You might enjoy dressing in an apron and cleaning. You might like baking, sewing or doing other mundane chores. Only to you, they're far from mundane!

I know one cross-dresser who has completely satisfactory experiences doing housework for his wife while he's dressed. All he does is put on her apron and gets to work. She has no idea that he's fantasizing about being her little slut while he does this. For him, wearing her apron turns an ordinary experience into a trip to paradise. To this day, Dan's wife wonders why her husband makes passionate love to her after tidying up. He doesn't feel compelled to tell her and that's fine. Someday, he might let her in on his little secret but for now, he's content to keep it inside. It's a wonderful story and best of all, it's true. I think it perfectly illustrates how to indulge in a fetish and still have a strong personal relationship.

What is your goal?

Many of you report that you enjoy dressing for long periods of time. You might finally end up masturbating but getting off isn't your ultimate goal. What do you like to do? Have you ever gone out while dressed? What was it like? Is it something you fantasize about or want to do?

Do you get into a submissive mindset when dressed?

You might like getting dressed within the context of a Dominant/submissive role-play situation. While this is similar to forced cross-dressing, the submissive frame of mind might be very different for you. Being forced often goes hand in hand with embarrassment. Conversely, being submissive merely means that you enjoy putting yourself into the hands of another. Which one of the above best describes you?

If you picture yourself as submissive while dressed, what do you wish for?

You might want your partner to tie you up, spank you or play with your nipples. Or you might want something completely different. Take a moment to consider your fetish "laundry list."

Chapters 12 and 13, which discuss Dominant/submissive interactions, will give you more help deciphering what you are looking for in this area. Remember to take notes right now to assist with your discovery process. Full disclosure will take time, however.

A Word about Cross-Dressing Academies

Although the focus here is on getting a partner to be comfortable enough with your cross-dressing fetish so that she will ultimately share it with you, there are some instances where this isn't possible. Either your partner isn't willing or you don't feel ready to disclose your penchant for cross-dressing to her. In cases like these, you may feel that you want to enact your cross-dressing "jones" with another individual, a professional of some sort.

In large cities like Los Angeles or New York, there are actually schools or academies which specialize in cross-dressing. One very reputable place I can personally vouch for is "Miss Vera's Finishing School for Boys Who Want to be Girls."

(www.missvera.com) Its dean is the very lovely Veronica Vera, who is both extremely capable and exceptionally compassionate. More and more, Miss Vera is sharing her knowledge with couples as well as individuals. Guidance on how to properly put on wigs, makeup and dress is given in an uplifting, supportive environment. She also instructs men and women on how to walk in high heels! Many of Miss Vera's students choose to learn how to dress as females purely in the privacy of their own homes while the goal of others is to go out on the town or to go shopping with "the girls." The choice is yours.

A bit of online research will probably reveal a host of possibilities in a city near you. Besides Miss Vera's Academy, a quick Internet search revealed places located in New New Jersey, as well as boutiques which cater to cross-dressers in locations like San Francisco, Oakland and Chicago.

In Summary

Your cross-dressing fetish is intricate. Use the headings I've listed above as a way to self-discovery. This is for your own personal exploration. Later, it will be useful if you choose to share your fetish with another person. Always remember that the more you understand yourself, the better you will be able to communicate to another.

Just so you know, women often find this particular fetish extremely confusing. They will immediately wonder if you're gay or a drag queen. They'll tell you it's a turn-off. They'll express concerns about what others will think. Most of all, they might warn you that sex while you're dressed is off the table. After all, she'll remind you that she's not a lesbian. If she wanted to be with a woman, she would have dated a female, she might even go so far to tell you. But be aware that much of this attitude stems from not completely understanding the nature of a cross-dressing fetish.

I'm not mentioning the negatives to frighten you or deter you from telling her. But rather, I'm sharing the possible opposition your partner might give to your cross-dressing so that you can have your information arsenal ready. Be prepared to fire back. It's not impossible to get your woman to participate in your cross-dressing fantasies. Be positive, confident and convey an attitude of self-acceptance. Don't be apologetic. When you accept yourself, she'll accept you.

I've personally met many women who eventually enjoy cross-dressing their husbands. They've developed a sense of humor and a relaxed attitude about their man's predilection. They understand that they are appreciated for being open-minded. Plus, they have husbands who are generous when they go on a shopping spree together.

You're not the only "woman" who enjoys getting clothes! If you go shopping together, always remember to get some items for your partner's wardrobe as well as for your own. I guarantee that the perk of beautiful lingerie, clothing and makeup for her as well as for yourself, ups the ante when trying to convince her to join with you in your cross-dressing adventure. Basically, she'll be thinking, "Now you're talking," and be ready to embark on the journey with you, high-heels and all.

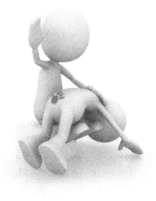

Chapter 10 - Are You An Adult Who Likes Spanking?

If you're an adult who has a spanking fetish, the Identification Process is particularly important for you. That's because spanking is a fetish that's misunderstood by most of the population. Tell someone that you like spanking and they might very well categorize you as some kind of pedophile. Unfortunately, most people are very uninformed about what it means to be an adult spanking fetishist. They don't get that it's a pleasurable, fantasy-based activity. They just recall their own personal terror inspired by the very thought of corporal punishment. The idea that you love spanking is inconceivable.

Let's be honest—spanking is a somewhat bizarre fantasy. This is because it's attached to negative childhood memories and the notion of punishment. But always remember that all fetishes are produced during the formative years. If you were born with the fetish gene, this environmental experience is then sexualized.

Spanking is something that most people were exposed to early on. Whether you were spanked or not, the idea of an adult spanking your bare behind is both embarrassing and frightening to a child. However, both fear and embarrassment are extremely stimulating within our brain activity. That's why the spanking fetish is particularly strong. It's also why most spanking fetishists are especially conflicted.

Somehow, spanking seems incorrect; the thought of being excited by something associated with children just can't be right, you reason. If you happen to feel this way, please remember to rethink and accept. Adult spanking fetishists are just that. You're an adult, and are choosing to engage in this behavior with another adult. Even if you're role-playing a childhood act such an aunt spanking a nephew or a teacher spanking a student, in reality, you're both adults. You're both playing a role, like the way an actor does in a movie. It's okay. Have fun with it.

Even pornographers don't get the concept of spanking. How many of you have been disappointed when you go to a spanking website that depicts women in leather flogging a naked male? That's a whipping, not a spanking. How many of you have felt ripped off by a DVD that has a naked female tied down and strapped until she's marked? That's a beating; not a spanking.

These days, there are many false, brutal images posted on websites that claim to be spanking-based but really aren't. A true spanking produces a pink bottom. It's done in the spirit of sensuality, nurturing or fantasy-fulfillment. Identification is necessary—and especially important—in the realm of spanking so you don't fall prey to societal misconceptions about spanking. You must identify your own spanking needs as a means of self-understanding and self-acknowledgement. This is necessary not only for you but essential if you choose to engage in your fetish with another person.

If you are an adult spanking fetishist, it simply means that you enjoy the act of giving or receiving traditional, over-the-knee spankings. Although this act is associated with childhood discipline, a spanking fetishist only exchanges spankings with consenting adults. Some of you might enjoy playacting or making believe you're in childlike situations such as a professor spanking a naughty student or a sexy neighbor spanking the young guy next door, but in reality, you're both adults.

Even if you like the idea of age regression and think about the kind of spankings you may have witnessed as a youth, you know the difference between fantasy and reality. In truth, you cringe at the idea of seeing a child get spanked in real life. Spanking as a fetish is an adult experience and these fantasies are always enacted between adult spanking fetishists.

As an adult spanking fetishist, you love to hear the very sound of the word "spanking" and you feel butterflies in your stomach by any reference made to spanking. You can barely utter the word without blushing beet red. You think about spanking when you least expect to. You see a pretty woman and wonder what it would be like to get a spanking from her. You notice a female in skintight jeans and feel an urge to give her butt a smack. (Remember it's an urge, not a reality!) Spanking is truly your cup of tea and the ultimate aphrodisiac. You just can't get it out of your head.

You weren't necessarily spanked as a kid but you remember being interested, deeply interested. You've wondered what it would be like to give or get a spanking ever since you can recall. Your curiosity about spanking grows stronger each day. You might see spanking as an appetizer but as a fetishist, it's more likely that you view spanking as the main course. If given the choice, you'd choose spanking over intercourse. In fact, you've never had an orgasm without some kind of thought about spanking. You never get tired of the idea of someone getting their pants pulled down and their bottoms spanked pinkish-red.

But as much as you love spanking, you're probably very confused about your fetish and constantly ask yourself why you like something so puerile, painful and nonsexual. You've spent hours wondering where your fetish came from but you can't come up with a definitive answer. Certainly, many adults were spanked as kids and most try hard to forget an event that was both painful and embarrassing. Why then do you relish it and obsess over spanking?

Most of you remember being exposed to some kind of spanking when you were growing up—either on TV (how many times did Ricky spank Lucy in "I Love Lucy?"), in movies (even G-rated ones like Elvis in *Blue Hawaii*) or in real life. You remember spanking as a "forbidden" activity. Spankings were given in private and were surrounded by secrecy, so that made you even more curious. Some of you might have heard screams, smacks and the sobbing of a sibling, friend or family member getting spanked. You wondered what it was like and you might have secretly been disappointed that it wasn't you. After all, though spankings seemed to be painful, the person receiving the spanking was also receiving a lot of attention. Because of this, your child brain might have made a positive association about them, something along the lines of: *Spankings = Attention*

All children crave attention and any kind of attention is better than no attention at all. Even if the attention comes in the form of a bare-bottom spanking.

Fear is also an aphrodisiac, and in your memory, there was always fear surrounding the act of spanking. That fear could later morph into excitement and feelings of arousal. The same goes for the curiosity factor. Spankings are a super-charged experience. Once again, there may have been an early connection between arousal and spanking. Adult spanking fetishists or "spankos," as they affectionately call themselves, have many theories or memories of early spankings. You may have guessed where you fetish came from but you don't know for sure. You only know how the act of spanking makes you feel. And that is very, very turned on.

There are many variables within the spanking community. The Fetish Checklist in Chapter 7 will help you pinpoint exactly what you do and don't like about spanking. The questions underscored in this chapter will help your response to be more pointed and detailed.

Do you think about spanking within the context of a Dominant/submissive (D/s) relationship?

You might like the idea of submitting to a spanking. To you, it's the same as submitting to a whipping or a heavy bondage session. You like the thought that your partner is having fun administering the punishment. You take the spanking to prove your love and devotion to them. To you, a spanking is romantic, and the red bottom you get as a result of it is evidence of your ardor for them. It's like a merit badge you've earned.

This mindset is very different than the mindset of a spanking purist. A real spanking purist acts as if they don't want the spanking, only they have no choice but to take it. Conversely, a D/s person embraces the idea of spanking as an act of submission.

If you are more of a D/s person, it's important to identify that. Please also refer to Chapters 12 and 13, which detail the intricacies of D/s relationships, to help you uncover the parameters of your fetish.

Are you a purist when it comes to spanking?

First and foremost, what do you imagine when it comes to spanking? Is the spankee bound or dangling over a knee? It's very important to make this distinction. If you like the idea of power exchanges or Dominant/submissive interplays, you can skip this chapter and proceed to Chapters 12 and 13 on D/s exchanges and male submissives. This only means that you're not a traditional spanking fetishist. You probably like spanking but only when it's combined with one person controlling another in a power play sort of environment.

If you're a traditional spanking fetishist, you focus on the idea of giving or receiving spankings. These spankings may be reminiscent of early childhood experiences but the interaction is, of course, between two consenting adults. The spankings may or may not be given for a reason. Sometimes the spankings are meted out as a kind of punishment. Other times they're administered as foreplay. Most often, the spankings are performed as a self-contained scene that is certainly arousing but not necessarily overtly sexual.

Are you a giver or a receiver?

Some spanking fetishists enjoy giving a spanking and consider themselves a "top." A top can also be referred to as the spanker. Others prefer to receive and call themselves "bottoms." Another name for a bottom is the "spankee." Still others like to experience a little bit of both worlds and therefore call themselves "switches."

Even if you've never participated in a real-live spanking, you can probably identify your chosen role. When you see a spanking photo, who do you identify as? Do you imagine the rush of causing someone to squirm on your lap? Or do you imagine yourself dangling helplessly over someone's knee?

Obviously, you should figure out where you stand if you decide to share your spanking fetish with another person. Some novice tops will opt to bottom for a while so they can get a sense of how to carry a scene. It's actually a good idea for you to bottom before you top. That's because you want to know what a real spanking feels like before you enthusiastically wail away on your partner's innocent, waiting behind.

Do you think about spankings as playful or punishing?

Like many fetishes, there's a spectrum when it comes to the kind of spankings that take place in your fantasy world. Some of you like to think about intense spankings given for the purpose of punishment. In this mode of thought, spanking is used as a form of retribution and correction. The person getting spanked doesn't want the spanking but in the end, they submit for their own good.

Spanking doled out as punishment takes on a life of its own. Somebody did something wrong. They're told that they have to be spanked. The spanker doesn't want to do it but there's no other choice. The person being spanked will protest, bargain, and beg. The spanking doesn't stop until a change in attitude has been affected. In a sense, the spankee is in control because if they want the spanking to continue, they simply don't have a change of heart—until their bottom has had quite enough.

You might also enjoy a spanking exchange that's more playful or fantasy-based. Though role playing spankings might be as painful as punishment spankings, they are still being administered within the guise of fantasy. It's not you who's getting spanked but the character who is. It's that willful shoplifter, that defiant truant or naughty cousin. The attitude in role-playing is more fun and lighthearted. Many of you love to read spanking stories. When and if you decide to play with another, you sometimes choose to bring some of your favorite scenarios to life.

The difference between a playful spanking and punishment spanking is not necessarily measured by physical pain as much as it is about the intent of the spanking. Playful spankings are more erotic or fantasy-based. Punishment spankings are about correction. Many adult spanking fetishists can get very serious (and specific!) about their spanking interactions. You have to determine your place on this spectrum.

Pay attention to your inner masturbatory fantasies. Think about the attitude of the spanker. Is she nurturing like a mom or stern like a school disciplinarian? Are the spankings given for reasons related to serious misdeeds or simply for naughty behavior? Most of all, do you imagine participating in spankings for real misbehaviors or just for make-believe mishaps?

Do you like spanking merely for the sensations?

You might like spanking simply because you enjoy the way that it feels. Some people find it erotic or pleasurable to be repeatedly smacked on the bottom. Hard, soft or medium? With the hand or implements? If you prefer implements, then which implements: a strap, hairbrush or cane? What material? Leather, plastic or wood? There are so many variations and so many specifics to identify.

You might also like intense sensations. The common term for this is masochistic or sadistic. If you identify with either of these categories, you are one who goes for the extreme. You enjoy giving or receiving spankings that are intensely painful. This distinction is very important for you to be aware of. It means that you will have to seek out a suitable play partner. This might seem more obvious for a top, but it's equally important for a bottom. Not every spanker is comfortable with playing hard. Some like it; others don't. Please make sure you are aware of your desires and then seek out a compatible playmate.

Some people find that a good spanking actually alleviates pain. Isn't that ironic? I've know people to say that a spanking reduces bodily stress. One spanko named Bobby even says that it helps with the agony of fibromyalgia!

Do you think of spankings as therapeutic?

Many people in the spanking community talk about spanking sessions in the same way others might talk about sessions with their counselors. They describe the release of emotion and tears. A spanking with a qualified top can actually help one get in touch with emotional pain. Some of you might envision talking about past or future feelings of guilt or regret.

Your hope might be that the spanking will help you to release deep, buried emotions.

While many report success with this type of "spanking therapy," always remember that it is an adjunct to working with a qualified therapist. The spankings might help you get to a breakthrough but ultimately, that breakthrough must be processed in a therapeutic setting.

Do you like the idea of going into subspace?

Many spankos talk about going into something called a "subspace" while receiving a spanking. This can be described as being a hypnotic trancelike state. The person goes deep into their own inner world. They lose touch with the outside work and feel very focused on themselves and on their bodies. As a result, many report having a cathartic release while they are in this hyper-intense emotional place.

Subspace is a very special state of mind. It must be experienced personally as opposed to being described. Generally speaking, the top should be experienced and qualified. She should know how to guide someone into this deep, intense state. For example, her pacing and buildup must be administered with care. Talking is kept to a minimum. Any sharp, unexpected smack or outside interference can disrupt the process. The spanking must be orchestrated with care from beginning to end.

While you might want to experience subspace, it's important not to make it the goal. Most people say that subspace just happens spontaneously. If you're curious about subspace, do include it in your Identification. When you play with another person, mention that you have thought about having this experience.

Is embarrassment part of the punishment in your spanking scenario?

In all honesty, the very act of a spanking is embarrassing. The idea of having to accept punishment is humbling and humiliating, the act of having your pants lowered or taking down your partner's panties. Maybe your spanking fantasy involves having to stand in the corner. Some of you even imagine asking for the spanking and admitting a wrongdoing in order to get spanked. I'm asking you to dig deep and look into what the idea of spanking actually means to you.

Don't be surprised if you're indeed turned on by the humiliation of a spanking. Humiliation is another fetish in and of itself. Spanking can be an embarrassing act…but an embarrassing act which is causing you to get wildy aroused.

Do you like the idea of a nurturing spanking?

Spanking is often seen as a nurturing, caring experience. Traditionally speaking, spankings are given for one's own good. Many of you love the phrase, "This hurts me, more than it hurts you." In fact, one of my clients referred to those very words being used in an old "Little Rascals" episode which aroused him to no end when he was a child. It's the segment when Spanky's father is getting ready to throttle his bottom. If you're a spanking enthusiast, you probably remember it…in exquisite detail.

Do you think about spanking as a means of behavioral modification or motivation?

Many people in the spanking community contemplate the idea of using spanking for the purpose of motivation. They think the idea of a spanking might help with losing weight, stopping smoking or cutting down on drinking. While the intent is good, in reality a spanking will not really get you to make a behavioral change. Nevertheless, it's an innovative method to take your fetish and use it for personal growth. Many spanking fetishists report that using their fetish makes dreaded activities more fun. It's a way to get your cake and eat it, too. As long as you realize that in reality, it's not the spanking but your own aspiration for transformation that will cause behavioral changes, it's fine.

Do you equate spanking with punishment?

Many of you do. After all, spanking is indeed traditionally associated with childhood punishment. That's where the idea of spanking originated. "Spare the rod and spoil the child," was once a popular credo. In truth, modern research has shown that spanking usually generates more negative than positive effects when it comes to disciplining a child. If it doesn't work for children, it certainly won't work for adults!

However, fantasies are not based in reason. You might feel that there has to be "a reason" for the punishment. Some fetishists in a spanking relationship purposely use "bratting" as a signal to let their partner know it's time for some spanking play. Basically, bratting is behaving like a brat. They'll put sugar in the salt shaker, tie your shoes together or even stick out their tongues. In other words, they create silly situations which give the go-ahead for a disciplinary or punishment spanking.

Some couples claim to have a domestic discipline type of relationship. This means that a husband and wife agree to use spanking for real situations that arise in the relationship. Spankings are administered for misusing the credit card, losing wallets and other irresponsible behavior. You might dream about such a relationship. Make note of it if you do.

I don't think much of the domestic discipline type of relationship. My own personal feelings about this sort of thing is that any fetish is based in arousal, not necessarily discipline. Fetish play works best when it's used to enhance sexual activity. Since spanking is a fetish which is derived from a very nonsexual situation, there is a temptation to spank for its original purpose, which was for behavior correction.

This is why I'm asking you to rethink that one. Would you really want to be spanked if you got a speeding ticket? Or bought something you didn't need? If you came home late, for example? Real-life situations must be handled in an adult way. Revisit using a sexual fetish for anything other than having a fun, arousing time.

Do you enjoy role-play with your spankings?

Role-play is a great way to get your desires met. It's a good way to get around the quandary of spanking for purposes of punishment and discipline. With role-playing, you can make believe you're getting punished for a real transgression. But of course, it's not you who's getting punished but the person you're pretending to be.

Role-playing allows you to bring to life your favorite spanking tales and fantasies. You and your partner can make believe you're different people in real-life situations: teacher/student, boss/assistant, aunt/nephew, sexy landlady/tenant. The possibilities are endless.

Role-playing allows you to get your spanking wishes met in a healthy, non-threatening way. This is not to say that people who enjoy Dominant/submissive play aren't naturally role-playing during their scenes, because they are. In reality, no one is superior over another but in that mindset, the submissive gives himself over to another person. It's similar to D/s interplay, but different. If you're a true spanking fetishist, you think about real people in real-life situations. Dominant/submissive role-play is more about caricatures: the lady in leather and her groveling slave.

Role-play is an excellent way for you to get started when and if you decide to engage with another person. In role-play, you create a comfort zone of make believe. It's not you who are naughty but the character you're playing. Role-play is a wonderful way to re-enact the fantasies you think about when you're alone. Many spanking fetishists use role-playing as the way they get to interact with others. It's enjoyable, arousing and provides an opportunity to get your needs met in a safe way that has established boundaries.

The attitude and severity of the spanking you give or receive is directly related to the role-play. Some role-plays call for sterner presentations while other role-plays are conducive to being more lighthearted. Role-playing can be very healing. It allows you to be re-parented by an authority figure who has your best interest at heart.

Some spanking fetishists are surprised that they'd even want to engage in spanking activities since it was a miserable part of their childhood. If that's you, take heart in the fact that you're actually doing something that is very healing for yourself. Re-parenting within the context of a spanking role play can be very powerful. You can get to be cared for, corrected but not abused. Always remember that a spanking is not a beating. Spanking is a loving expression of real care and nurturing.

Do you like to age regress?

You might fantasize about spanking in its original context. A mom, aunt or teacher puts a younger person over their knee. In reality, that's not what you want to do but your fantasy is your fantasy. Please don't feel guilty. You're not really focusing on a child getting spanked. Most likely, you're putting yourself in the place of the child or wondering what it would feel like to interact with the sexy spanker. This is where the public gets confused about the fetish but I want to make sure you're crystal-clear about this. There's a huge difference between fantasy and reality because many spanking fetishists love the idea of age regressive fantasies but recognize the line between fantasy and reality.

If you like the idea of age regression, role-play is the way to go for you. This way, you can re-enact your favorite fantasies with another consenting adult. You are both grown-ups playing make-believe. See the difference? It's important for you to know and be clear about this. This way you won't be ruffled if someone accuses you of fantasizing about children. You aren't. You're fantasizing about spanking and the spanking situation. It's an essential concept for you to grasp so you can come to terms with your fetish in this important Identification Phase.

What are your favorite spanking positions?

Most spanking fetishists favor the traditional over-the-knee position. Even then there are variations. Do you prefer the use of a straight-back chair or a stool that allows for a feeling of helplessness? Or do you like couch-spanking for comfort? Do you also require scissoring between the legs so movement is impaired? These are all important spanking aspects to consider.

Sometimes a spankee might prefer to be spanked in the bent-over position. Generally speaking, bent-over spankings are conducive to punishment spankings administered with an implement like a hairbrush or a wooden spoon. Many people like to have a combination. Think about what you like and then convey the message.

Do you like the over-the-shoulder carry fetish along with your spanking?

The over-the-shoulder carry fetish can be a fetish in and of itself. It's when you throw your partner over your shoulder or when she does this to you. Again, there are elements of power exchange here. I know of a number of spanking fetishists who like to combine their carry fetish with spanking .They fantasize about the idea of swatting the behind of the person they are carrying or vice versa. If that happens to be you, please note this in your Identification Process.

Do you imagine incorporating implements into your spanking play?

Spanking implements are props used in conjunction with spanking fantasy play. They are not whips, hawses or floggers. They are implements associated with the idea of punishment. You might envision hairbrushes, paddles or belts and wonder what they feel like. Well, you don't have to wonder any longer because any and all of these implements can be incorporated into your spanking scenarios. The beauty of it is that they never have to be used beyond what you or your partner is comfortable with.

I remember one spanking fetishist who reported to me that his first spanking was almost his last. Why? Because he had a fantasy about being spanked over the knee with a hairbrush and that's exactly what his partner did for him. However, she had no experience with spanking and didn't realize that hairbrushes got their reputation for a reason. They hurt! Especially when not used correctly or too harshly.

Remember, you can fantasize about whatever you wish but proceed with caution when using these implements. It's best to err on the side of gentleness. You can always adjust the severity of a spanking the next time. Adult spanking is not usually about causing pain unless that's what you specifically seek.

What spanking verbiage triggers you?

Think about the words that trip your trigger. You might have certain phrases that are music to your ears. What word combinations do you like? I know many adult spanking fetishists who love to be told, "You just earned yourself a good spanking!" or "You won't sit comfortably for a week!" and "Get over my knee. Now!"

Identify the phrases that have particular meaning for you. If you engage with a partner, it will be important to communicate this information before you get down to business.

Do you have a preference for special costuming, clothing or uniforms?

You might fantasize about a specific role that calls for a particular type of uniform. Policeman, fireman and French maid are all possibilities to enhance the play if that's your thing. If you like to age regress, you might choose to dress accordingly.

Many of you might find it stimulating to be spanked wearing an outfit reflective of the scenario you're enacting. You might then want to don the uniform you wore to Catholic School or Boy Scouts, gym shorts or khakis.

Some of you have very specific tastes about outfitting. In fact, the craving is so strong, it could be considered a secondary fetish. Tight jeans, pantyhose, rubber pants or girdles might come into play here.

A number of adult spanking fetishists are very particular about underwear since traditional spankings are usually administered progressively: over the clothing or on top of underpants until the spanker works their way toward the bare bottom. Panties are very important to male tops. They might have a preference for certain types of underpants such as slutty lace or see-through. Even color can play a role. Many spanking fetishists like old-school, full-back, white cotton panties. How about you?

Do you have a dual spanking fetish?

You might have something very specific that goes hand-in-hand with your spanking fetish. The specifics I've seen include but are not limited to: a need to only be spanked on diapers, tight hose, a specific brand of jeans or rubber panties. I call this a dual fetish because unless the specifics are present, you will not reach satisfaction. Do you have a dual spanking fetish?

In Summary

The spanking fetish is one that is complex and has many facets. It's never enough to say that you just want to be spanked. You must be able to describe the position, the implements and verbiage you enjoy hearing. You also have to differentiate between a punishment and a playful spanking. Before you communicate, it's helpful to answer the many questions posed in this chapter.

There also might be something else I haven't touched upon that's important to you. Remember to include it in your initial inventory and subsequent communication. There's no such thing as too much information. Nobody's a mind reader. Fetish is very specific by nature so remember to figure out the key components that meet your own individual requirements.

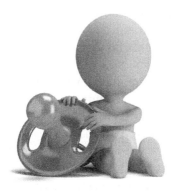

Chapter 11 - Are You an Adult Baby?

If you enjoy the idea of reverting back to your first year on earth, you have an infantilism-based fetish. In other words, you like being an adult baby. There are many components to this fetish so it's important to identify where you lie on the infantilism spectrum. This spectrum can be as simple as wearing adult diapers or as complex as living as a baby for a significant period of time (one hour or an entire weekend, for instance). If you are an infantilist, you probably relish the thought of being fed, changed and fussed over.

I know this is a hard fetish to accept. You've questioned your desires and tried your best to put them to rest. Yet, like all fetishes, its draw is strong. How do you describe the comfort you feel in diapers? Or the joy you experience being played with? Or the thrill of being powdered when your diaper is changed? You have a highly-misunderstood fetish. It's the butt of many jokes. Infantilists are portrayed as silly, freakish and just plain weird. Yes, it's a bit unusual but that's all it is.

Society at large doesn't understand the basic tenets of infantilism so you have to contend with a slew of falsehoods and myths. First and foremost, you're seen as being unmanly. The truth is that you can be very manly. Just not in the moments you're pretending to be a baby.

Then there's the awful misconception that you want to play with babies for sexual gratification. This is absolutely untrue. You do not sexualize other infants; you only sexualize yourself as a baby. You don't want other babies in the picture because you're the baby. This is an important concept for you to understand and verbalize. You might have to verbalize this if you are ever the object of ridicule.

Infantilists are portrayed unkindly. They're joked about and made fun of in movies and TV shows. It's a difficult fetish for most to imagine. As a result, it's ridiculed. Case in point, Octomom Nadya Suleman was cast as a "mommy" in an adult fetish movie. People loved pointing their finger at her. The actor in the film was over the top as well, as was the movie itself. Nobody took into account that infantilism is a real fetish that real adults happen to have.

It's not easy having an adult baby fetish. Even you might consider it pretty outrageous when you stop and think about it. Yet, sometimes being an adult baby is what you like. A lot! Transforming yourself from an adult into an infant literally takes your breath away. The concept of regressing backward in time is appealing, exciting and erotic to you. It's also something you're compelled to do, drawn to. Many of you have been practicing infantilism on your own for years. It's a solitary activity and a relaxing way for you to spend time alone. But sometimes it feels lonely. I bet you wish you could share this experience with another human being.

The idea of sharing your infantilism fetish probably feels incredibly daunting, too. Who would understand this? You barely get why you like what you like yourself, so how could you expect someone else to get it? And the "why" isn't as important as the fact that you do, that your fetish exists at all. You're constantly beating yourself up over it.

But I want you to stop. Stop feeling guilty about your fetish. Remember that fetish is imprinted into your sexual makeup in the first few years of your life. It's here to stay and at this point, you have to begin accepting that it's a part of you, much like a fondness for chocolate ice cream. The better your understanding of your fetish, the deeper your self-acceptance will be.

Because being an adult baby is a very tough fetish for you to grasp, it's hard to try and explain to another person. Sometimes the very thought of disclosing your adult baby wishes to someone else might even paralyze you with fear. I wonder if you've ever lied about it.

One of my clients did just that. The first couple of years of his marriage, Brian wore diapers to bed. His excuse was incontinence. He actually got away with it for a while. He lied to his wife about his "condition" and gave her phony medical reports. One day, she called his bluff and made him go to a urologist of her own choosing. That was the day Brian contacted me. He decided that he had to finally own up to his fetish. My advice to him was not to make a rash decision. Before Brian spoke to his wife, I asked him to go through the same Identification Process that you'll be starting soon. The reason I asked Brian to hold off? I wanted him to understand himself before attempting to communicate his desires with another person.

Like you, Brian had to figure out the motivation behind his fetish. He had to figure out if wearing diapers was a solitary activity or one that he would like to share. It was necessary for him to identify if there were any connections to humiliation or Dominant/submissive interplay. He also had to figure out how much information he wanted to reveal to his wife. Obviously, he was caught in a lie but ultimately he still had choice about disclosure. Full disclosure or partial disclosure is a big decision.

Ultimately, Brian chose to admit that he lied about having a medical condition. After the Identification Process, he realized that he did in fact fantasize about having D/s interaction and even disciplinary fantasies in conjunction with his fetish. Brian decided to wait until a later date to share that aspect of his fetish with his wife. He acknowledged that she first had to deal with the fact that he had lied. That, he agreed, was a big deal. Next, he had to admit to having a complex fetish.

Sharing so much heavy-duty information with his wife would take time. Brian and I agreed it was imperative that he take her feelings into consideration and give her ample time to digest what he was telling her. Doing a thorough investigation through an in-depth Identification Process later proved to be extremely helpful to Brian.

For now, you recognize that you fall under the spectrum of the infantilistic fetish where you enjoy the idea of being an adult baby. You probably have recollections of this fetish that stem way back to some of your earliest childhood memories. It's amazing that even little infants can be aroused. If you believe the genetic theories about fetish, it may be that you have a propensity toward being aroused by stimuli outside the conventional. Environmentally, there was something about being changed or fussed over that gave you a sexual charge that later became a point of arousal for you.

Right now, you have a vague idea about what you like, but I'm asking you to pinpoint your triggers and dig deep. The answers lie within your masturbatory fantasies. If you aren't sure of the response to any of these questions, always reference what you think about when you are alone. Try to recall the websites you frequent and their slant. Some infantilism fantasies go hand in hand with the idea of Dominant/submissive role-playing. Others fall into the category of humiliation, embarrassment and being forced.

Your Identification Process is necessary for you to understand yourself. It is essential if you choose to share your fetish with a partner. You can't communicate what you don't understand. Take some time to identify the parts of this fetish that have particular meaning for you.

These questions will help guide you through the Identification Process:

When did you first realize that you had a need to regress?

Most fetishes form early in life. Think about when you first noticed that you wanted to regress back into "simpler times." Was there any catalyst? Was there any life-changing event you can connect to this desire? Many times, people act upon their fetish when they're feeling stressed. There's a strong link between anxiety and fetish. The infantilism fetish is all about self-soothing; it comes from a very nurturing place. So, please be thoughtful and try to get in touch with your own anxiety levels. In other words, how does your fetish help you when you're feeling uptight?

Are you an adult baby or a diaper lover?

Adult babies enjoy everything to do with being a baby. Do you like the idea of being fussed over? Tickled? Picked up? If you participate by yourself, you might be doing some of these activities already. Perhaps you even have your own baby bottle, pacifier or rattle. You might have set up a special place to indulge yourself. Perhaps you curl up in a soft blanket, read baby books and suck your thumb. Can you imagine doing these activities with another person? Would you enjoy having your partner join in and participate in your fetish? I know it would make you feel extremely vulnerable, but being genuine will lead you down the road to true intimacy.

If you're a diaper lover, this means your main arousal point is wearing diapers. There's something about this that feels oh so good. You might like the way they hug your hips, encase your bottom or brush against your penis. It may feel like you're wearing a security blanket. It's very comforting.

You also might like the idea of wetting yourself and then being changed. If this is the case, what do you like about it? Some fetishists say they like the sensation of warm liquid running into the diaper. Others like the feeling of freedom it gives them. Still others report that they like the idea of being mischievous or naughty.

Do you also enjoy defecating in your diaper?

If so, what do you enjoy about soiling your diaper with feces? Could you imagine having your partner change you? If the answer is "yes," what do you think her attitude would be? Would she just change you as though she was your mother and pooping in a diaper was expected behavior of a baby? Or would she be more stern and admonish you? What type of reaction would you want her to have?

Does your diaper fetish have to do with control?

Part of being a baby is linked with total dependence on another human being. Do you like the idea of being dependent on a caretaker? Do you crave not being able to do anything at all? Now's the time to identify any and all of your feelings about the idea of losing control as a baby. Is this idea of control something that resonates or holds true for you? Can you imagine sharing your fetish with another human being or is this something that you are content to do when you're alone? What kind of attitude would your imaginary caretaker have? Would she be nurturing? Strict? Matter-of-fact? Would you like the idea of being at her mercy?

Are you a bottle or breastfed baby?

Are you an adult baby who likes to get your nourishment through the nipple? If so, you might be sporting a bit of a dual fetish with female breasts. Often, one fetish connects to another. Identify if breastfeeding is part of your fantasy world. But perhaps you like the idea of being given a bottle. Maybe you've already been feeding yourself. Can you imagine having a partner hold the bottle for you? What would this be like?

What are some of the props you currently use or would like to incorporate into your fetish play?

All right, we've covered the notion of baby bottles. How about rattles and pacifiers? Would you enjoy playing with baby toys? If so, what kind of toys? Can you imagine yourself inside a crib? Crawling on the floor? Being bathed?

Many infantilists have very elaborate setups to indulge their fetish. What do you imagine having? If you could have your ultimate fantasy, would it include a baby room? If that's the case, describe it. Do you imagine being in your nursery alone or with your partner? If you would like to share your fetish with another person, this Identification Process will be most helpful when it comes to communicating your needs.

What kind of diapers do you like?

You might have a preference for disposable diapers, cloth diapers or rubber panties.

Do you also like to be spanked?

Some adult babies like to be punished for wetting. The

punishment is often a light spanking over the diaper or on a bare wet or bare dry bottom. Again, there is often an overlap with fetish fantasies. What kind of a spanking do you imagine yourself getting? What is the role of your spanker? Is she a nanny, a mom or stern caretaker?

Do you enjoy some humiliation with your fetish?

Humiliation is another key component in identifying your fetish blueprint. At the heart of the infantile fetish might be a need for humiliation and possibly degradation. Your fetish actually helps you to acknowledge this aspect of you without letting it get in the way. Infantilism gives you an outlet. You have a time and place to feel this way and you do it on your own terms. And you've found an arena for you to enjoy the humiliation rather than fight it. Good for you!

In your fantasies are you being laughed at? Made fun of? Being called names? What are your own dark, humiliating thoughts concerning your fantasy? Is there anything someone could say that would be hurtful or counterproductive?

When you identify the fact that you like humiliation with your baby scene, it's important to also know your limits. Is there anything your partner could say that would be a complete turn-off and ruin the scene for you? If so, write it down. It's important to communicate what you like as well as anything you don't like.

Do you want to be "forced?"

The notion of forcing someone to do an act against their will happens with other fetishes such as foot worship, cross-dressing and bisexual acts. If you like to be forced, it means that most likely, you enjoy this within the context of some type of Dominant/submissive role-play scenario. Basically, the concept of being forced takes the fetish act out of your hands. There's a sort of comfort in feeling that regression is something you're made to do rather than want to do. Someone's making you wear a diaper or suck your thumb. It's out of your control. It's in someone else's hands. You have no choice. Yet you do.

Is being an adult baby part of a Dominant/submissive role-play?

If so, then "Mommy" replaces the Dominatrix. Mommy is still the dominant female, the one in control, but her persona goes directly to the source: mother. Mom is your first experience with rules and boundary-setting.

In this kind of fantasy power exchange, do you imagine incorporating other kinds of D/s play such as bondage, tickling or spanking? You might request a variety of acts or you might be totally focused on being made to be a baby. Only you know what goes on inside of your mind. Your fantasy belongs to you. Your fantasy is unique.

Are you an exhibitionist?

Many adult babies like the idea of being seen. It's a turn-on that your partner is witness to your regression. Exhibitionism often goes hand-in-hand with humiliation or embarrassment. It's key to identify if being seen is a component of your baby fetish. Take note of it so you can communicate it if you choose to do so.

Are you a sissy baby?

Some adult babies like to cross-dress, too. This means you not only want to regress to being a baby, but you want to be a girl baby. How does this affect the way you're treated? Are you fussed over even more? Or are you ridiculed for being a sissy? What significance does cross-dressing have in your fantasy life? How would it affect a scene with your partner? Don't forget to mention girly clothing, dolls and other props that might be necessary for your scene.

If you'd like to have your partner participate, what would be her role?

You must figure out if you want her to be an active participant or an observer. If she's a participant, what role does she play? You might be an adult baby who's seeking a nurturing mommy. To that end you will want her to be there, loving you in a variety of ways that only you can prescribe. She might be there cooing, tickling or feeding you from her breast. You might imagine her changing your wet diaper or playing a game of peek-a-boo. Perhaps you're subconsciously seeking the loving mommy you never had. That's why I'm asking you to do the soul-searching prior to communicating your requirements to your mate. Only you know what you need and want.

You might also seek someone who's more strict or disciplinary. To that end, your mom will be more like a Dominatrix or an authority figure. She will set rules and punish you for disobeying. She might spank you for wetting your diaper or for being fussy. Again, think about the kind of mommy you're looking for and the inclinations you have. Some adult babies secretly want the strict but loving mom they never had, a good mother who's direct and sets boundaries. She will reward you when you're good but punish you when you're bad.

In Summary

Not only is your fetish unique but it's also unique to you. The Identification Process is designed to guide you through a journey into your inner fantasy life. It's meant for you to solidify your thoughts about your fetish. It will also help you to know your triggers and the essential components of your fantasy. Only by doing a thorough investigation will you have a real understanding of what your fetish entails. Only by obtaining this knowledge can you effectively communicate it if you choose to do so.

Your fetish is just one component of the person you are. Though you enjoy fantasizing about being a baby, this doesn't make you any less of a man. You are, in fact, courageous in the sheer act of being able to take an honest look into yourself and acknowledging an important aspect of what makes you tick.

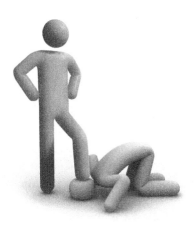

Chapter 12 – Are You into Power Exchanges?

If you identify with being either Dominant or a submissive, it means that you are adventurous and enjoy trying on new roles for size. Traditionally, men are the ones who are expected to be in control while their female counterparts are thought to be more compliant. But that isn't necessarily the case. These days, we're more flexible with gender expectations though traditional values still hold true. As a result, many males find Dominant/submissive (D/s) exchanges to be a healing change of pace.

If you're a fellow who enjoys D/s, your fetish is played out within this arena. For you, it's not only the fetish, but the mindset that goes along with it. You enjoy fetish play within the context of Dominant/submissive parameters. Plainly speaking, your fetish is attached to the idea of being in charge or relinquishing control.

For example, you are ordered to engage in fetish play or you want to be the one to give the commands. In that vein, a foot fetishist who's into D/s exchange not only wants to worship feet but he also wants to be ordered to do so. The guy who has a tickling fetish and identifies as a Dominant, will love the idea of his submissive losing control beneath his fingertips. Likewise, the guy who has fetish for female bottoms may enjoy viewing them while being smothered by a commanding female. So, with D/s, it's not only about the fetish, but it's also about exchanges of power. The fetish then becomes a part of something larger.

For some, the fetish is actually all about control. Who has the power? Who doesn't? If you identify as someone who is primarily interested in power exchange, you probably envision a dungeon-like setting. There, the dominant is the "top" and in control. He or she performs a variety of acts based upon the desires of their submissive or bottom. The main fetish is the dynamic between a top and bottom. You can see how that's very different than those of you who have a specific fetish for a body part, fabric or act.

Power exchanges allow for creativity. You get to try on a new persona for size. You get the opportunity to spread your wings and be someone else. Or you get to capitalize on the attributes you already possess. For example, someone who has trouble making decisions can now make the most of that trait. You're no longer prodded with, "Make a decision, then live by it." Instead, you get to lay back and put yourself into someone else's capable hands. As my client Floyd, so aptly describes it, "Sometimes you just want someone else to do the driving."

If you have tendencies toward leadership, being a top allows you to take charge of someone else completely. Of course, these exchanges have boundaries and are controlled. The interesting thing is that even though the top appears to be the decision-maker, in reality he or she is catering to the whims of the bottom. The submissive almost always calls the shots. The Dominant takes the lead but is directed by the bottom. Everyone has aspects of the top or bottom within them. D/s role-plays allow us access to these traits. In the dungeon, we can get in touch with either role. We can be more of who we already are or take on a role that's the opposite of the way we're usually seen.

If you fantasize about submissiveness, you long to let go. People used to equate submissive men as high-powered business executives who needed a break. While this old idea may hold true for you, in our current world, many men are getting in touch with their softer, more feminine personas. Therefore, the submissive role is becoming easier to connect with no matter what you do in real life.

Women's roles are also changing. It's commonplace now for women to take on lead roles in action movies and to be given executive roles in the boardroom. We're getting used to seeing women in positions of strength. As a result of seeing women take on non-traditional roles, many men feel comfortable about getting in touch with their softer side. They discover that it's fun to submit to that sexy bitch dressed in latex, leather or a business suit.

You've seen her, the Bitch Goddess, in comic books, feature films and in adult movies. What would it be like to submit to her bidding? To suffer for her pleasure? To do what she bids no matter how degrading or humiliating?

And if you're the one on top, how do you see yourself? Are you commanding? Are you sexually demanding? Do you imagine instructing her about how to pleasure you? Or do you wish to sexually tease her until she begs for release? D/s fantasies are complex and will be very specific to what you find arousing. In the world of fantasy and fetish, anything goes as long as the exchange is between two consenting adults.

Now it's time for you to identify what aspects of D/s power exchange resonate with you. The following questions will guide you:

Are you a top, a bottom or a switch?

This is, of course, the obvious question but it's your starting point. I think that deep down, you know what you like and it's your task to communicate it simply and directly.

If you like to top, you must pinpoint what it is you enjoy about control. Do you love the idea of your lady being as timid as a Geisha girl — sweet, subservient and obedient? Or do you enjoy taming the feisty shrew like Bianca in Shakespeare's play? Mindset is important and something you should articulate.

How do you imagine yourself as a top?

Are you fatherly, a brawny superhero or an even-tempered

business exec? Think about the kinds of scenes that get you going. What kind of Master do you want to be?

You have to take into account that your fantasy is only a fantasy. When engaging with another person, you need to set limits. A newcomer who isn't into this scene will be a more challenging participant than choosing a female who's already in touch with her own submissive nature. The latter person is certainly an easier choice but sometimes the person with no experience also excels because the two of you can set the parameters for a relationship that would work uniquely for both of you.

What do you like to do when you top?

Some men just like to tell their partner how to dress and behave. You know, order her to wear a skintight skirt without panties. Or command her to touch your penis discretely at the movies. Others like to give step-by-step fellatio instructions. You don't want anything too extreme. You merely relish the idea that you're the guy calling the shots.

Most tops do wish to engage in some kind of Dominant scene where bondage, flogging or spankings come into play. If your partner is a novice, you must be very aware of her lack of experience and possibly, her lack of enthusiasm, for your scene. One Dom I know spanks his non-scene girlfriends "lighter than light," as he phrases it. He's perfectly content stripping his girlfriend naked, placing her over his lap and tapping to music on her bare behind. He still gets the aura of control but his lady is happy and doesn't feel exploited.

As a top, your most challenging task will be to get your non-scene partner to want to engage in domination games with you. In this day and age, many women have an aversion to being in second place. They view kowtowing to a male as antiquated and Old School. They might also envision S/M interactions as something cruel or violent.

Lucky for you *Fifty Shades of Grey* has made Bondage and Discipline a household term. The book trilogy focuses on the romance between a lifelong male top and his non-scene girlfriend. How can Christian Grey get Anastasia Steele to enjoy the rigors of heavy-duty dungeon activity? The answer is, he doesn't. Christian's extreme approach is immediately problematic to his young but very confident girlfriend. However, through trial and error, communication and deep love, the couple eventually comes to a workable compromise. The fact that it takes them three whole novels to reach an effective agreement emphasizes my point that introducing a non-scene partner to your fetish is never easy. However, it can happen with commitment and patience.

I personally enjoyed the *Fifty Shades of Grey* trilogy because it opened the door for many non-scene men and women to consider alternative sexuality choices. The fact that the books were huge best sellers with women is an encouraging sign that the times they are a-changin'.

Do you like to bottom?

I know you've been raised to think that the male is supposed to be the leader, the guy in charge. And you might very well have that role in the workplace. But in your sexual headspace, you love the idea of being taken. Of having a woman order you around and take complete control. Yes, it conflicts with what social mores have told you, but remember, your fantasy is your fantasy. You like being a submissive. Period. End of story. So, how do you convey this idea to a partner and still keep your dignity?

Luckily, you've already done your homework and have arrived at a place of acceptance. You don't have to justify or defend what you like. This happens to be your turn-on. That's reason enough to indulge. You enjoy the idea of female dominance and you refuse to apologize. Confidence is key here. You absolutely must be confident or you'll lose your lady's respect. The more positively you discuss your fetish, the more eager she'll be to participate.

Don't forget, many women already like the idea of being on top. They've been fighting for equality for decades! They've struggled for a power position in the workplace and on the homefront. The opportunity of being in control is a no-brainer. You're offering her something fun and out of the ordinary. She's going to love this and it's your job to "sell" the idea to her. Enthusiasm is infectious.

When you're explaining your fetish to your non-scene partner, remember to take it slow. Don't divulge too much information at once or you could overwhelm her. Introduce her to the concept of domination. Gently educate her and explain what you're after.

What's your Dream Dom?
Do you fantasize about a fictitious Dominatrix who sports leather or latex in a dungeon-like setting? Is she a sexy temptress or cruel sadist? You might even have a penchant for a more domestic type of disciplinarian, like a frumpy, cranky housewife. (Think Harriet Nelson in a bad mood.) If so, you might be looking more for a mommy or a nurturer who has no choice but to straighten you out with some good, old-fashioned discipline.

Again, the mindset and your fantasy go very much hand-in-hand with what you must communicate. Remember, saying that you want her to dominate you is not enough. You need to be specific and explain precisely how you want her to top you and what you want her to do once she's assumed the role. Some male submissives enjoy serving a "Goddess." This means, kissing her perfect bottom, licking her boots, sucking her toes, and so on. Others want more elaborate types of dungeon activity like physical restraints, toys and whips. Or maybe you want a retro, over-the-knee spanking. Only you have the ability to supply the adequate information to make your fantasy a reality.

Are you a switch?
Again, it's not enough just to say that you'll be the top or the bottom. How are you going to do that? People known as switches like to top AND bottom depending on their mood. Others like to switch back and forth while doing the scene. You whip me and then I'll whip you. I'll instruct you on how to pleasure me and then you instruct me on how to pleasure you.

More on Switching

Switching is healthy!
You might not have considered the idea of switching because I know many of you see yourself as one role or the other. But I'd like to add some encouragement about switching within the

context of a long-term committed relationship. The reasons are outlined below, then we'll go back to a few remaining items to consider in your Identification Process.

Switching is great for a potential top.

There's no better way to teach a novice Dominant than by having her go submissive first. Rather than instruct her verbally, you get to demonstrate exactly what you want. She'll know precisely what the implements feel like so she'll be more aware and cognizant of the pain she will eventually mete out. You can also demonstrate attitude, verbiage and tone of voice to her if she subs. When it's her turn to be "woman on top," she can mimic you and be the kind of Dom that really gets you going.

In the realm of BDSM (bondage, discipline, sadomasochism), many professional Dominatrixes are required to be submissives first. This way, they really get to understand what it feels like to be tied up, clamped or whipped. In turn, they will be more compassionate toward their bottom.

If one has never been tied up themselves, they won't understand that eventually the ropes will cause joints to go to sleep and tingle. If one has never gotten clamps on their nipples, they might be inclined to leave the clothespins on too long because they're unaware of how the pain builds to a crescendo. Part of being a Dom is to be caring toward your submissive. Switching will give you and your lady an appreciation of and true understanding of both roles.

Now, back to a couple more important areas to consider in the Identification Process:

What kind of costuming and equipment do you have in mind? Unless you're going the professional route, you'll have to supply the equipment and all of the other accouterments necessary for play. This would include costumes, accessories and paraphilia. It's better to have them available and ready for her to use. Don't expect her to go shopping on her own! Remember she's new to this and it's your job to show your appreciation for her involvement by making this as easy and as non-stressful as possible. Besides, you'll enjoy the anticipation as you prepare for the event. On top of that, you'll be sure to get the tools and outfits you like.

What type of verbiage is key to your scene?

As with all fetish scenes, communicate specific verbiage you like and the tone of voice in which you like it delivered. Do you prefer her to speak quietly, shout or sneer? The more you tell her, the better the scenes will be. Never forget to share favorite images, clips and photos so she can get a better visual or what you are seeking.

In Summary

Power exchanges which are about Dominant/submissive role-play are at the core of many of your fetish fantasies. Before getting into the specifics of what your fetish fulfillment entails, it's necessary to clarify whether or not your fetish is performed within the context of Dominant/submissive play. Spell out the details of your role but also be open to switching as a way to broaden your own sexual horizons, demonstrate what you like and develop more understanding of the other person's role.

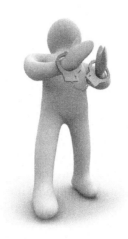

Chapter 13 – Are you a Male Submissive?

You might have a fetish which is played out within the context of a D/s relationship. Many fetishes happen to fall under the realm of Dominant/submissive role-play. This means you require something special that's not always associated with traditional sex. This is the fetish part of the piece.

Being a male submissive also means that you imagine having your fetish fulfilled within the guise of being dominated. You want someone else to take lead. You like the idea of letting go and relinquishing control. Your fetish fulfillment is now in the hands of another individual. Instead of having freedom of choice, you are commanded to participate by your Superior. You have no alternative but to obey her wishes. Inside, you imagine complying because of a wish to please or a fear that you will be punished. Either way, fetish fulfillment is out of your hands and driven by someone conceived to be more powerful than you.

On the other hand, your fetish might actually be submissiveness, not the domination aspect of the puzzle at all. Your fetish is to be submissive within the context of a D/s relationship. Whatever transpires is secondary to the fact that your fetish is to serve another person. You like the idea of total abandonment of responsibility and having someone else hold the reins. You enjoy the ritual of thinking about your top as a beautiful Mistress or Goddess. To that end, you simply like the idea of serving, pleasing and pampering your lady.

You're inclined to view women as the superior race (at least within the context of your fantasy world). You are open to any of the sadomasochistic acts associated with dungeon play. Those would include but are not be limited to whipping, flogging, spanking, bondage, cock-and-ball torture (CBT), nipple torture and trampling. You might also be open to foot or leg worship, sissification (also known as feminization) and other humiliating acts which are mutually agreed upon with your top. While you are participating in these S/M activities, they are secondary. The primary wish is to be at the mercy of your top.

One client of mine named Carl enjoys the concept of Female Dominant (Fem/Dom) exchanges. To date, he has not expressed his interest to his wife of three years. However, Carl has an ingenious way of getting his yearnings met. Often on the weekend, his wife prefers to lounge in bed and do absolutely nothing. Opportunity knocks! Carl indulges her wishes by volunteering to do the cleaning and other household chores. Lucky wife! She's happy to make a list while he hands her the TV remote. As she's resting, Carl's diligently working. All the while, inside his head, he's fantasizing that he's her slave. Lucky Carl!

In fantasyland, Carl has no choice but to obey his Mrs.'s wishes. He's motivated because he wants to please her. Mundane tasks like scrubbing the toilet now bring on joy and arousal. When Carl's done, he returns to the bedroom and buries his tongue between his wife's legs. He's extremely aroused and she has no idea why. She happily enjoys the ride.

Although it's a win/win situation for both Carl and his wife, it's still bittersweet for him. He doesn't like the idea of keeping secrets from her and feels that honesty is the key to intimacy. One day, he hopes to be truthful about his eagerness to do her bidding but he doesn't feel quite ready yet.

Carl is currently in the midst of doing his Identification. It appears that his primary desire is to serve, please and pamper his wife. His secondary needs include various acts of humiliation. On one end of the spectrum is foot worship and at the other end of the spectrum is cuckolding (playing the role of a husband with an adulterous wife). By identifying these wishes, Carl will be able to figure out what to share with his bride based upon importance.

For example, Carl feels that his wife will probably be agreeable to forced foot worship. On the other hand, cuckolding is a more complex fetish and one that would be difficult for any newcomer to deal with. How important is it to Carl? As it turns out, his Identification Process revealed that cuckolding is indeed more of a fantasy than it is a reality. Carl isn't even sure about that himself so it's not necessary to bring it up anytime soon. If ever.

You're probably reading this chapter because you have a fetish that is ideally enacted with a dominant partner. You should figure out if it's the fetish or the D/s relationship that's most essential to you. Those with a very strong fetish will probably figure out that it's the fetish you couldn't give up.

Imagine that you're a person with a dual fetish for mohair sweaters and domination. You might have a dilemma—what's more important, the sweater or being dominated? If it's the sweater, then you identify yourself as a mohair sweater fetishist, because in truth, domination is secondary to the object of your desire. On the other hand, if you think more about being dominated and the sweater is merely a prop or image, then you would probably be happy to give the sweater to Goodwill. The distinction between being a pure fetishist or a submissive is essential during the Identification Stage.

Identifying the specifics will clarify who you are and lead to thoughtful self-knowledge. The following questions will help usher you through the Identification Process. Answer them honestly in order to arrive at a better understanding about yourself and your role as a submissive.

Do you have one particular fetish? If so, what exactly does your fetish entail?

Though this question is basic and you can say you know your fetish, write it down anyway. Note whether you have one fetish or several fetishes within the context of being a submissive male.

How do you imagine your fetish being fulfilled?

Write down how you have been achieving fetish fulfillment to date. Is it solely through fantasy during masturbation? Do you also get satisfaction from viewing images online or watching video clips?

Have you ever engaged in this fantasy with someone else?

If you have a fantasy for D/s exchange, there's a chance you might have seen a professional Dominatrix. Think about your experience/s. What did you enjoy? What aspects could have been better?

If you had to give up one aspect of your fantasy, would you feel compelled to hold onto your basic fetish or would you prefer to be dominated by a top?

This is pretty much what Mohair Sweater Guy had to decide. It wasn't a hard choice for him, though. He clearly had a strong need for mohair sweaters in his life. He was very happy to have his wife don a sweater during relations. It was an easy decision for him.

On the other hand, the fellow who liked humiliation along with D/s had to deeply ponder his decision. In the end, for him, it was more about D/s than the hankering for a specific humiliating act like cuckolding.

You must give this question a great deal of thought. Only you can make this choice. And remember, when all is said and done, it might not even have to be a choice.

How do you define yourself as being submissive? What does it mean to you?

The very term "submissive" can have totally different meanings to different people. There's probably no single term to describe exactly who you are but the standard definition of a submissive states that you are a person who willingly conforms to the authority or will of another. You might be described as being obedient, compliant and generally passive. I realize this definition is negatively based and I apologize in advance. It's society's definition, not mine. I have better ways for you to think about it.

To me, a submissive male is actually someone who is very loving and enjoys pleasing his partner. The typical sexually submissive man is bright, capable and successful. Carnally-speaking, he simply enjoys following his partner's lead. He likes being attentive, caring and actively displaying the loving side of his sexuality.

In many ways, I believe that a submissive male is more evolved. He's not afraid to be in touch with qualities that are generally thought to be feminine. Are you sensitive, attentive and easygoing? If you have these traits within the context of bedroom play, then you're probably sexually submissive. Some of the following lead questions might help you define and communicate what being submissive actually means to you.

Are you submissive by nature?

Unfortunately, we live in a global community which has very rigid standards when it comes to gender identity. Women are the ones who are supposed to be docile and yield to the opposite sex. Men are thought of as the strong ones. Throughout history, men have been perceived to be the leaders. They're often characterized as being strong, powerful and aggressive, but in truth, many men don't fit this stereotype.

At the end of the day, we're all multifaceted individuals. As it turns out, whether or not we are passive or aggressive has less to do with our gender than it has to do with our own personal genetic and environmental factors. DNA, birth order and family history weigh in much greater than male or female factors. Today, we're finally recognizing the strength, power and intellectual capabilities of women. In turn, we are also recognizing the softer, emotional and more traditionally feminine aspects of men. As a result, many men are now happy to declare themselves submissive. Perhaps you are one of them.

You might just be submissive by nature. You are more comfortable in, and in fact, flourish in an environment that is structured and planned out. You do your best when you're given guidelines and direction. You don't mind authority and truthfully, you're rather comfortable with someone else in charge. This doesn't make you any less of a man. Instead, it makes you invaluable because you know how to offer support and dependability within the work environment.

Today, you're also aware that your submissive nature spills over into the bedroom. Dynamic, confident and forceful women turn you on. When it comes to being sexually pleasing, you'd rather give than receive. You also prefer being told what to do as opposed to second-guessing what someone else has in mind.

Finally, you have an outlet that not only recognizes your natural submissive inclinations but actually supports them! Within the D/s relationship, it's not only your role to be compliant; it's your actual duty. You are rewarded for following orders and punished for noncompliance. The scene actually encourages you to enhance your tendencies.

What a refreshing change of pace for men who have tried hard to be something they're not. A D/s scene actually exaggerates the roles of the person who's in charge and the person who's compliant. The Mistress calls the shots and the slave obeys. No more having to justify, explain or feel bad about your natural inclinations. You enjoy the scene because it encourages you to be exactly who you are. And that guy is loving, sweet and wants nothing more than to please his partner.

What's so bad about that?

Are you sexually submissive as an escape mechanism?

The classic idea of the male submissive has to do with the law of opposites. For many years, it was said that most male submissives were attracted to the lifestyle because they were high-powered business executives looking for a break. That guy might be you. The theory was that submissive males were under a lot of pressure and were always having to make decisions for others. (Remember Floyd's comment from the last chapter about wanting someone else to do the driving?) As a result, the idea of a female leather Mistress was exciting because it offered escape.

When the traditional male/female roles are reversed, you get to take a breather from reality. If you can relate, then you're probably a guy who's used to being in control. You would like the idea of being a submissive but only in a very specific way, with established boundaries. You can get into the head space for a specified amount of time. It's exciting to let go. However, generally speaking, once you orgasm, the mindset instantly disappears. You climax and you go back to being the stereotypical, high-powered guy that you are.

Please be aware that these submissive mindsets are not absolute. They really fall into a spectrum. It's important to deeply consider your response to this question so you can communicate better about who you are. You'll also have a better sense of the type of woman you'd like to seek out. If you're a laid-back guy you'll do better in life with a more assertive, organized woman. But if you yourself are a control freak who even likes to control his D/s scene, look for a partner who is more compliant and there to please you, whether or not she's dominant or submissive by nature.

Do you like the idea of D/s play as a lifestyle?

Again, if you are a natural submissive, you will want to choose a more dominant partner. You'd probably like to be able to incorporate some aspects of the D/s scene into your day-to-day life. While I'm not a proponent of rigid roles or living a D/s lifestyle full-time, you might enjoy a lady who's able to get into the role because, like you, she is the role. Rather than get angry when you're sprawled out watching the game instead of doing the dishes, it might be fun if she just yanked you over her knee for a quick spanking. When she's stressed out, she might love the idea of lying back, spreading her legs and having you service her. And you'd be more than willing! What a fun life.

Are you more of a compartmentalized player?

If you fall on the dominant side of the spectrum in your daily life, chances are good that to unwind, you want your D/s activity when you're so inclined. It wouldn't even feel amusing or enjoyable to have your lady threaten you with a whipping unless you were in the mood. You prefer to play only when you're turned on and feel like being subservient.

If this is the case, it's okay. You just have to communicate that to your partner very specifically. There's nothing worse than having your partner misunderstand her role. Basically, you like her to be dominant only at the right time, place and when the mood is right. Otherwise, you prefer your partner to be herself. Someone whose personality and values are compatible with yours. After all, you might love steak, but you don't want to eat it every night, correct?

How does your submissiveness translate to your role in the bedroom?

Since we're discussing sexuality, it's important to understand how you have come to define yourself as one who is sexually submissive. It might mean that you'd simply rather your lady take the lead when it comes to bedroom activities. This has the added attraction of being a turn-on for her as she gives you exquisite details about how to please her. She would be able to vocalize exactly how and where she wants you to touch her. She could teach you her erogenous zones and guide your fingers to provide optimal pleasure. As a dominant type of woman, she'd have no trouble giving you instructions on sexually satisfying her both orally and genitally through intercourse.

Being sexually submissive in the bedroom doesn't necessarily have to lead to any kind of kinky or fetish type sex. Though sexual submissiveness is generally linked to fetish, it doesn't have to be that way. You might simply enjoy a more aggressive woman. Unfortunately, even with that tiny variance, our society may have made you feel a bit embarrassed and ashamed. Hopefully, you've been able to reframe that way of thinking and realize that being sexually submissive actually makes you the true stud. Why? Because you take the time to find out what your woman wants, you listen and then you please her to the best of your ability.

To make sure you understand the role of sexual submissiveness and fetish, I'll dive more deeply into the dynamics here before I continue with the questions to help with your Identification Process.

Sexual Submissiveness and Fetish

Many fetishes lend themselves to the idea of a dominant female taking lead. She either guides or "forces" the submissive to bend to her will. Of course, nobody ever forces anybody to do anything they want to do. But within the context of your own individual fantasy construct, there is a degree of having no will of your own.

You might be someone who enjoys one fetish and one fetish only. Or you might be a person who gets excited by giving their partner a "laundry list" of acts you would perform within the context of a Dominant/submissive role-play scenario.

Since this is the chapter about general submissive play, let's explore some related fetishes commonly associated with interactions between a dominant woman and a submissive male.

Back to the Identification Process:

Do you like strap-on play and anal intercourse?

Many men are aroused by anal play. They simply like the sensation of being penetrated anally with a finger, butt plug or dildo. Even though some might perceive this as an act of submission, it's only submissive if that's the established mindset of the play. Again, you must ask yourself if it's the idea of anal stimulation or is it anal stimulation performed by a superior female within the context of D/s role play that you crave.

If you like anal intercourse, what goes through your head when it's occurring?

If you are a true submissive, you might like the idea of being penetrated anally because of the role-reversal aspect. The female is not only taking a lead position but she's also visually sporting male genitalia. This image might make you feel very docile and wanting to serve and please. You want to bow down to this dominant person to demonstrate your submissive nature.

Imagine a dominant female dressed in thigh-high boots, a leather bikini and brandishing a big, strap-on dildo. For some, this visual takes their libidos to a new level. And for you, the visual just might be enough to push you over the edge. You might be a submissive who just likes to see their partner dress in this type of dominant attire. If so, then it's definitely the image of a woman wearing the strap-on that gets your motor running. In all probability, you could most likely forego the D/s exchange aspect of the fetish.

Do you like giving fellatio?

Is the idea of sucking a dominant woman's "penis" or dildo appealing as a way to demonstrate your compliant nature? Oral sex is traditionally a submissive act, especially when one is on the ground with their face being straddled by the other. If you are naturally a bottom, you'll enjoy performing the act of sucking her dick. It doesn't mean you're a homosexual. Not at all. You clearly want to be with a female. You just get turned on being in a submissive role.

If you want to feel the dildo penetrate you, what's your mindset?

Someone who has a strap-on fetish is driven by sensation. Once the dildo is inside it stimulates the prostate gland and feels sensational. If you like the feeling of being penetrated, then you have a strap-on fetish. Your primary desire is for your woman to sport the dildo and pierce your anus.

You're into D/s if you have submissive thoughts attached to your fetish. You want to be taken by your Dominant. You want to lose control. You ache to feel more like a woman. Consider your mindset about strap-on action. Your fantasies are key in helping you understand whether or not you are indeed primarily into D/s.

Do you want to be "forced"?

The idea of being forced is very different than merely wanting to take on a submissive role. If you think about getting forced, it means that you're doing something that you and your partner conceive of as humiliating. In truth, you want be penetrated. But part of your fantasy is pretending that you don't. I know this sounds tricky but take pause to figure out your personal motivation for wanting to be "fucked."

It's important to know this because your partner will need to adjust her own attitude and persona accordingly. The idea of being forced means that you're getting reamed as punishment, for purposes of embarrassment and ultimately, because your partner wants to. Your fantasy is about non-consensuality, though in reality, it's completely consensual, even orchestrated. You're merely role-playing your own internal fetish.

In this role, your woman must be commanding. Remember to disclose the verbiage you think about when you masturbate so that she can heighten the encounter. The more you reveal, the better the experience will be.

Are you primarily a foot fetishist or a foot fetishist with a desire to submit?

Men with foot fetishes are fairly common. Often, it has nothing at all to do with being submissive. The foot fetish is such an intricate proclivity that I've dedicated a whole chapter to the variables associated with liking female feet. I've included foot fetish here as well rather than only in Chapter 8 because it sometimes goes hand-in-hand with Dominant/submissive role play.

Do you think of yourself in a subservient place when interacting with the female foot?

Many submissives like the idea of incorporating some kind of foot worship within the context of a Dominant/submissive role-play. Getting down on your knees, kissing, licking and caressing your Dominant's shoes, boots or bare toes might merely be an important warm-up to other acts.

However, if you like to perform foot worship as one of many duties in the dungeon, you are not technically a foot fetishist. Instead, you are someone who likes to incorporate some kind of interaction with your Dom's feet in conjunction with other D/s dungeon activity. Which is perfectly fine; it's just different than a standard foot fetishist.

Do you like to cross-dress?

There are a variety of reasons you might like to dress up in female clothing as a male submissive. You could enjoy the feel of the material, the way you appear in the mirror or you might just like the naughtiness of wearing "forbidden" garb.

However, if you view cross-dressing as an act of contrition, humiliation or punishment then you are someone who enjoys cross-dressing within the context of Dominant/submissive interaction. Being ordered to don panties, stockings or transform into a female is very different than doing the act by yourself. When you enjoy the idea of cross-dressing in order to please or submit to a dominant partner, it means that you view dressing as a submissive act. This is an important distinction that needs to be articulated to a potential play partner.

What's your mindset about cross-dressing?

If you see cross-dressing as a submissive act, it means that you want to dress in order to be pleasing to your Dom. Deep down, it's what you want, but within the realm of your inner fantasy, it's the wish is to dress in order to be pleasing to your top which is your chief motivator. In other words, she wants you to do this; not you.

You picture being her female slut, toy or lady servant. Or you imagine that dressing is a form of punishment. Because of a transgression, you are commanded to dress up and be her female servant or maid. Only you know what you think about when you're in this mindset, so it's your duty as a bottom to clearly communicate your specific inclinations to your top.

Do you imagine being forced to cross-dress?

Within the sphere of a D/s cross-dressing role-play, your fantasies might include the idea of being "forced." This means you view cross-dressing as something embarrassing or humiliating. While you like dressing, it's really the concept of embarrassment that gets you going. You know, you have to perform an act that you would never do on your own. But no matter how repugnant you find it, because you are a submissive, you are committed to do the very things you imagine are difficult or even impossible.

The tenets of a D/s relationship require you to "face your fears" and go to places you might find abhorrent. However, when you are in the throes of a D/s encounter (sometimes referred to as a "session"), your sexual nature comes to life and is open to particular acts you wouldn't normally want to do. You allow yourself to experience things you previously only fantasized about. Your top essentially gives your id (the part of the mind in which innate instinctive impulses and primary processes are carried out) permission to do the things your self-critical superego would never allow.

Do you enjoy pain or do you enjoy pain as a part of your submission?

Masochists enjoy sensations of pain. Phrased another way, they enjoy intense sensation and pain happens to be one of them. Just like some people like extreme sports, the masochist enjoys extreme pain. If you are a thrill seeker when it comes to receiving pain, it by no means classifies you as a submissive. You are merely a person who wants someone to inflict pain on your body. The relationship aspect of being a submissive is pretty meaningless for you.

Real submissives don't necessarily like pain. They will, however, receive pain if they feel it is pleasing to their dominant partner. Taking pain is a submissive's expression of love. You receive it because she wants to give it. Of course, like any fantasy, it's ultimately you who knows the kind of pain that is sexually stimulating to you. Some might like a wide variety of sensations. The thought behind it is that whatever your partner enjoys doing to you is what you enjoy.

Conversely, you might be someone who's more specific about the dose of pain they like. Perhaps you enjoy being whipped but not slapped. You might like cock and ball torture but hate having your nipples touched. You could love to worship a leather body but bare feet are a turn-off. Only you know what you like, dislike and the combinations that float your boat.

Do you have a specific fetish that's associated with D/s play?

If you have a fetish that requires another to mete out pain, you probably think you're a submissive who should seek out a D/s relationship. This might be true for you. However, it might not.

There are a number of fetishes that do require interaction with another but the mindset does not necessary have to be about D/s. It's important for you to figure out where you stand on this crucial issue. Attitude and mindset will be extremely significant if you decide to communicate your fetish desires with another individual.

Here's a partial list of fetishes that produce pain. What context is most arousing for you?

Spanking

This is a fetish that was commonly thought to be under the guise of D/s, but in reality, it's very different. Most adult spanking fetishists think of themselves as being naughty or worthy of punishment. However, they don't view themselves as being subservient.

Those who enjoy a sound spanking from the submissive vantage point like the idea of submitting to the sensation. They might be partial to that type of pain (sharp, hot, stinging) and to pain on the buttocks region, but they also like the idea of the spanking as an expression of losing control.

Nipple Torture

Do you love having your nipples played with, squeezed, pinched or even tortured? Again, consider your mindset. If it's the sensations, no matter how severe, you have a fetish for nipple torture. But, if you imagine being subjected to pain for your lady's pleasure, then you are a D/s fetishist. Though you prefer to have the pain limited to your nipple region, you still choose—and have a need for—the role-play associated with D/s interaction.

Bondage

You might like the idea of physical restraint and being rendered helpless. But if the restraint itself has meaning attached to it, this signifies that you like bondage as a part of the D/s experience.

Think about what bondage means to you? . Why do you like to be restrained? What is it that you find so attractive about losing control? Would you enjoy being tied up and left alone? Or, do you fantasize about the idea of being restrained in her quarters (i.e. a dungeon or bedroom), under her control?

Once again, it's important for you to identify whether or not you like bondage for the sake of bondage or if it is part of the overall D/s experience?

Other fetishes that can stand alone or lend themselves to D/s interaction:

So many fetishes can be performed for the sake of the fetish or they be seen as an expression of submission. A true submissive imagines partaking in whatever act his Dominant wishes to carry out, no matter how repugnant it seems. Of course, you will disclose your preferences to your dominant partner beforehand but your mindset is to please her. It means you would endure a spanking at her hand because it pleases her to do so.

Notice how this contrasts with a spanking fetishist who enjoys being spanked under the guise of someone who is naughty and deserves punishment. Or someone who would allow their partner to torture their nipples because she finds it fun rather than the fact that you enjoy stimulation to that part of your body. They're the same acts but just have very different motivations.

This leads to the Big Question during the Identification Phase:

- Are you a submissive or a pure fetishist?

Ask yourself what's your mindset about your fetish? Do you imagine it performed in a dungeon-like setting by someone you deem as your superior? Or do you want all of the emphasis on your fetish and on your fetish alone? If you had a choice, would you keep your fetish or relinquish control to your dominant partner?

Think hard about this decision in conjunction with any fetish I've mentioned. I'm listing the most common ones here, in alphabetical order, so yours is easier to locate. If yours isn't on this list, I apologize. But the question can remain the same even if your fetish isn't listed.

Here goes:
- Body worship
- Bondage
- Casting
- Cock-and-ball torture
- Cross-Dressing
- Electricity
- Farting
- Forced eating
- Medical
- Nipple torture
- Piercing
- Smothering
- Spanking
- Tease and denial
- Toilet slavery
- Trampling
- Whipping

Points to keep in mind:

Be clear in your Identification Process.

Because only you know, you absolutely, positively must be clear about what you want. If you like whipping, be specific about the implement. Do you like a flogger, a single-tail whip, a riding crop or the combo platter?

Corporal punishment might be your preferred dungeon activity but do be specific. Is it an over-the-knee spanking you crave? A bent-over paddling or a caning with restraints?

If you enjoy bondage, what do you like to happen when you're all tied up? At that pivotal point, do you want your nipples touched, clamped or teased? Do you want your penis and testicles tied tightly with weights? The possibilities are endless.

I realize that many of you have never experienced any real, live D/s interactions. However, think about what excites you when you're fantasizing and masturbating. What do you picture a Dominant doing to her submissive? These are the activities you should ascertain. Only then can you share them with a partner if you make the decision to do so. When you're communicating to another person, let her know your level of experience, of course. This must be shared with your top.

Safety First!

A good top will be cognizant of your limits. She will provide you with a safe word which allows you to communicate without breaking the scene. Ultimately, you are in control of what you do or don't do. But within the parameters of your fantasy, you might want to imagine that you're out of control. Verbal or physical cues which are established prior to play will allow your top to know if the pain is too much, too little or just right for you.

Nothing breaks the mood more than a feeling of dissatisfaction. Ironically, many submissives get frustrated because their partners are too cautious. They're afraid of hurting you. But as frustrating as this might be, erring on the side of caution is much safer. A simple code phrase like, "Mistress, I deserve a much harsher beating," might be just the ticket to letting her know she can drop the kid gloves and go to town on your bottom. It's important to establish a way to communicate when you want her to step up the pace as well as bring it down.

In Summary

If you are a male submissive, you are faced with many challenges. First and foremost, you have to get to a place of understanding that your role is valid. Though it might go against the way you were programmed to think as a man, the submissive male is actually extremely evolved. You are a human being who is more in touch with his gentler side. Sexually, you want to experience relinquished control and give yourself over to another person. You want to allow yourself the pleasure of being a dynamic, totally-rounded individual.

As a submissive male, you don't have an agenda in quite the same way as someone who has a very specific fetish, but rather, you are open to all kinds of experiences. You are willing to try almost anything—within the context of your own personal boundaries, of course.

Remember to go through the Identification Process for

yourself first. The initial step is in figuring out if you are a pure fetishist or a person who has a fetish that would be performed within the context of a D/s relationship. Once you make this distinction, you will know how to proceed. Your Identification Process will be instrumental in helping you communicate your desires to a dominant play partner.

You just might discover that what's most important for you is the idea of interacting with a dominant female. This D/s interaction is indeed your fetish. You might have a preference for specific acts or you might have a secondary fetish, but your primary fetish takes place in the dungeon. You are man who gets aroused by following orders, testing limits and being unconventional. Roll with it!

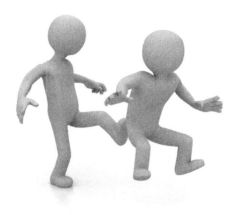

Chapter 14 – Are You into Humiliation?

The idea of being sexually aroused by derogatory situations, words or events is indeed baffling. You wonder why in the world you get off on being teased, embarrassed or degraded. How come it's extremely exciting for a beautiful woman to tell you that your penis is too small? Or that she wants to make love to a "real man" while you watch? That you're not good enough to kiss her shoes? Why would you want to be leashed, collared and paraded around like a dog? Or be forced to call yourself a sissy? It makes almost no sense at all. Yet, you identify as someone who has a fetish for humiliation.

Although this fetish is associated with D/s exchange, it may also stand alone. For example, you might like the idea of the cuckold fantasy without any of the other sadomasochist accouterments. Or you might relish the embarrassment of having to strip naked in front of two or more clothed women. These women are simply females. You don't identify them as "dominant females" per se.

Many men who like D/s power exchange consider themselves to be "lowly toilet slaves." But a fetish for golden or brown showers might just be the rush you get from being urinated upon or shat upon. You don't want to be "commanded;" you just want to be humiliated.

Humiliation fetishes are not necessarily about control. For you, humiliation might purely be about experiencing something out of the ordinary, getting in touch with your fear or pushing your limits. Only you have the answer. Making this distinction is an important aspect of your Identification Process.

It's not unusual to use coping mechanisms in order to deal with unpleasant events. For example, victims of rape do something called "splitting," where they actually leave their bodies while the event takes place. They report feeling like they are floating outside of themselves as a way to distance themselves from the violation.

Rescue workers and first responders also have an unusual way to cope with a critical event. They often employ humor as a way to ease the tension. Some may see this behavior as inappropriate, but in truth, the humor is a much-needed distraction.

Maybe you were bullied by your peers or treated badly by your parents. These events can have a catastrophic influence on your emotional growth and development because you unconsciously learned to lose trust and view your environment as unsafe. Abuse is something that many families consider to be shameful. Therefore, you don't tell. You learned to keep your secrets to yourself. Yet, the body remembers the trauma. You carry it with you every day and as a result, navigate through the world being hyper-vigilant or defeated. Many are not even aware of what an enormous effect these past events affect their present.

Did you know that acting upon humiliation fantasies can be healing? That's because you're acknowledging a part of yourself that most people try to repress or hide. You're acknowledging the embarrassment that's already there. By expressing your inner shame, you actually experience cathartic release. Exaggerating these fears within the context of a fantasy setting, allows you to experience the absurdity of your fears. It's like taking these feelings out of yourself and putting them into a box: you don't deny their existence but you don't have to carry them around in your daily life.

By bringing the "skeleton out of the closet," you diminish the power these feelings had in the past. Now they have a place, and that place is within your sexual makeup. These feelings don't define who you are. They're merely fantasies that can be fulfilled at the right time with the right person (hopefully, your mate).

When enacting a fantasy that might be trauma-based, your partner must be cognizant of the potentially-sensitive nature of the scene. Old feelings might be triggered. And that's okay, as long as you ultimately trust and feel safe with your partner. A great deal of communication before and after the scene is essential. The scene just might help you to release old hurts and shame. Many describe feeling euphoric after experiencing a true emotional release.

Don't say you like verbal humiliation without being specific. And also, be careful what you ask for.

Make sure you're not like Jim, one of my clients who wasn't specific about his desire for verbal put-downs—and got much more than he bargained for and experienced serious repercussions. What Jim wanted was to be teased in a generic way...nothing too personal. Jim enjoyed hearing phrases like "worthless slut" or "cum receptacle." It never occurred to him that he should disclose specific verbiage to his partner. Big mistake. Jim's wife went for the obvious and made fun of his weight. This was not fun for Jim because the insults hit too close to home. Being called a "fat pig" was hurtful instead of humiliating because Jim was indeed overweight. The poor guy became upset and totally lost his feelings of arousal. His wife also felt bad because she didn't want to hurt his feelings; she just wanted to fulfill his humiliation fantasy.

To avoid mishaps like this, your Identification Process must be precise and thorough in order for you to communicate effectively if you eventually choose to do so. These fantasies bring out your vulnerabilities so proper verbiage, attitude and enactment is crucial.

The following questions will help you identify your sexual triggers and define what humiliation means to you:

Are you into humiliation in conjunction with a D/s relationship?

Many people who consider themselves as "tops" in the D/s community will naturally assume that some kind of verbal or physical humiliation must be incorporated into the scene. That may or may not be effective, and in truth, the top should ask her bottom if he's into humiliation at all. For now, you have to figure out which is more important—the D/s interaction or your fetish for humiliation.

Do you like verbal or physical humiliation?

Verbal humiliation is about words or verbiage. Most of you can probably rattle off a number of key words or phrases that cause your penis to stand at attention. Verbal humiliation might take the form of being jeered at. I know of many men who find it arousing to be told that they have a tiny penis. Supposedly, even Howard Stern! It may or may not be the truth. Nevertheless, there's something you find highly exciting about being ridiculed.

Physical humiliation is about having to do something that you might find embarrassing. Examples of physical humiliation would include being leashed and collared, holding exposing positions, or having to masturbate in front of others. You might also dream of wearing silly outfits, doing a strip tease or being a human ashtray, all for the sake of being amusing to your Dominant counterpart.

Physical and emotional humiliation can be expressed by many different acts or words. Identify yours. For each of these fetishes, please include any special verbiage, costuming or props you require. Below, I've compiled a list of the specific fetishes and questions specific to that fetish.

Do you like to be farted on?

If this is your thing, remember to identify the circumstances. Do you like a woman to hover over your face? Fart into your mouth? Do you want to be forced to smell the gas? Is there any verbiage that will enhance the experience of being humiliated? Remember that those of you who have a farting fetish like the thrill of the forbidden. If you enjoy the D/s aspect you might like the "forced" aspect of the farting fetish.

Do you like golden showers?

What are the circumstances you like being urinated upon? Where does this take place? What's the scenario surrounding the scene? Do you imagine swallowing the urine? Does she say anything during the event?

Do you enjoy brown showers?

What are the circumstances you like being shat upon? Where does this happen? What's the storyline? Does she say anything while she does it?

Please take note that in the event of golden or brown shower fantasies, don't discount the idea that your fantasy can indeed turn into a reality. While the thought of eating real excrement can be much different in fantasy than it is in reality, there are ways to get this fetish met. Some guys will substitute brownies as a yummy alternative to human excrement. Thickened brownie batter can look very much like poop.

Other brown shower fetishists will have their partner give herself an enema first. Then, when she's completely cleaned out, she will give herself another enema. Some men find the clean water shooting from a woman's bottom very stimulating...maybe even you.

Do you like being smothered?

The humiliating part of smothering is getting your air supply cut off. In a D/s relationship, the woman controls your breathing. However, if you just like being smothered, you might actually enjoy the fact that you are underneath your woman's buttocks and that she's sitting on top of you in a superior position.

Do you like the idea of forced masturbation?

Yes, this definitely goes into the D/s mindset but you might just like the idea of exposure. You might fantasize about being told to masturbate in front of a group of women. Another variation would be about deprivation. I.e., you're not good enough to have sex with so you have to make her orgasm. After she's satisfied, you're allowed to pleasure yourself—or not. There are all kinds of variations here. What are yours?

Do you think about being degraded?

Being slapped in the face? Spit upon? Being forced to eat or drink something that is disgusting? While many enjoy TV shows like "Fear Factor" that are captivating, like watching a train wreck, some might find this example of overstepping to be exciting. Especially if the person pushing the limits is a Dominant female. Again, these scenes might go hand in hand with your D/s fantasies but they might also stand alone. Identify the meaning they have for you.

Do you enjoy being stepped on or trampled?

The image of a man being stepped on like a piece of carpet is indeed humiliating. This fantasy goes hand-in-hand with the feeling that you are worthless. Once again, the actuality of having someone step on you will help you to get in touch with the absurdity of the situation. Do you really deserve to be stepped on? Hurt? Of course not! But somehow, saying that you do and actually enacting the fantasy takes away the power of self-hatred. It demonstrates how just how absurd self-hatred is.

Do you have a cuckold fetish?

The cuckold fetish addresses the feeling of not being worthwhile enough to please your woman. Therefore, you want her to have sex with another man, possibly even someone who is well-endowed. You watch her receive the pleasure she can't experience with you. This fetish characterizes the ultimate in humiliation for many men.

In truth, you may or may not want to ever turn this fantasy into reality. Some fantasies are better left as fantasies. You might just like the idea of watching your woman the same way you enjoy watching porn. If you have hidden bisexual fantasies, you might also be curious to see what it looks like to be with another man. My opinion is that this fantasy is one that would only work in a relationship that is long-term, with a couple who are experienced D/s players. It could be very tricky emotionally otherwise.

Nevertheless, your fetish is your fetish. Identify exactly what aspects of cuckolding turn you on. What kind of a man would you want to see with your wife? What does he look like? What's his penis like? Be explicit in your Identification Process.

Never forget that your wife can always verbalize your fantasy—she can describe it to you instead of actually doing it. I know one couple who did just that. Her husband would often have her tell him stories about the various men she would meet on her lunch hour. In truth, she was always dutifully at her desk, but her stories made for some very steamy sex while his fetish needs were acknowledged in a manageable way.

Do you think about forced bi?

Though many fetishists feel anxious about having bisexual thoughts, the idea of forced bi is not about homosexuality as much as it is about degradation. How terrifying for a straight guy to be forced to turn gay. Don't make the assumption that he's being forced to do what he wanted to do anyway.

Many of you like the idea of humiliation as a challenge. What can be more challenging than being forced to do the very thing you shirk from? Again, forced bi is a more complex fetish since it entails another human being. These wishes can also be met verbally by your partner describing the details of a fantasy encounter to you. Identify the particulars of your fantasy so that you can communicate them clearly to your partner if you so choose.

Is spanking something humiliating for you?

Some men like the idea of spanking as humiliation. It's the association of being treated like a child—being forced to take down your underpants and bare your bottom. Is this the way you feel?

Do you like to be told to strip naked?

There's an entire fetish dedicated to the idea of naked men and clothed women. It's often referred to as CFNM. The fantasy stems around the idea of being forced to disrobe. Sometimes you imagine being naked with your wife, one-on-one. Often, you might think about being naked among a group of women. Imagine being the naked husband at your wife's all-female book club? I know, it's not likely to happen but once again, it makes for fine masturbatory material. It would also be an easy story for your wife to tell you while you're playing with yourself.

RCR

You may have noticed that I admitted many of your fantasies might be difficult to bring to light. And that's perfectly okay. In my book Sex, Fetish and Him, written for the woman who wants to understand—and help fulfill—her man's fantasies, I describe something called an RCR. That's short for Relax, Come and Relax.

Basically, RCR means you masturbate while your wife talks to you about your fetish. During the self-love session, you pleasure yourself to the brink of orgasm, then stop and relax, then start up again. You can take your penis in hand or your wife can, then massage you to completion at the very end. It's a much more intimate way to masturbate because your wife actually gets to be a part of your fetish world by actively participating as your own private erotic storyteller and/or masseuse who gives you a "happy ending. "

In Summary

Humiliation is another vast umbrella term that houses more specific fetishes. Often, they come about as a result of sexualizing trauma. Though this would initially seem like an unusual way to deal with unpleasant memories, in truth, bringing these fetishes to life or expressing them in masturbatory storytelling is a very healing exercise. You are releasing the bad feelings that many hold inside. This catharsis gives way to a sense of relief. These verbal expressions of low self image are given a place to exist, are compartmentalized, and therefore, don't have to rule your life. You give them a voice but it's strictly on your own terms. Ultimately you take back the power and control, which is a very good thing.

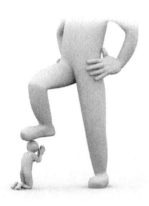

Chapter 15 - The Less-Common Fetishes: Off the Beaten Track

This book is not meant to be an "encyclopedia of fetishes." While I devoted several chapters to specific fetishes, I did so in order to provide examples of how to apply the Identification Phase of the Five-Point Fetish Plan. These chapters can all be adapted for you to use, no matter what your fetish is. With that said, I know what you're thinking:

> *"Sure Jackie. Easy for you to develop a Five-Point Fetish Plan and tell me that I can feel okay about fetish. While that might work for someone with a simple foot fetish, it will never work for me. My fetish is so peculiar that I can't even find a website that captures what I think about during masturbation. You don't get it. I'm doomed."*

But I believe that no fetish is too complicated. No fantasy is too outrageous, wild or crazy. Never forget that fetish is a fantasy. It's something you think about which provides a feeling of sexual arousal. I'm well aware of the fact that some fetishes require intricate settings, materials and skill in order to fulfill. I'm also aware that in reality, some fantasies are impossible to capture real time. That's because fetishes often live inside our heads. They are daydreams or imaginative events. They are impossible to recreate. But that doesn't mean you can't enjoy them.

While it's true that some fetishes might be more unique than others, my Five-Point Fetish Plan can work for anyone. Even you. That's because the crux of the Plan really isn't about the specifics of your fetish, but how you perceive your fetish in general. If you view your fetish as weird, you'll feel weird. If you tell yourself you're odd, you'll feel odd.

On the other hand, if you recognize that your fetish is different, develop a sense of humor about it and realize that you have many special qualities besides having a fetish, you'll feel just fine. In fact, you'll feel so fine that fetish will not get in the way of developing an intimate relationship. It's all how you think about it. And I want you to think of fetish as a small quirk, as a fantasy that's unusual and creative. It's not sick. You're not sick. You're simply the man that you are. With a little something extra.

The Universality of Fetish

Every man who has a fetish feels different than other men. These feelings of being different are often interpreted in a way that triggers depression, anxiety and self-doubt. It doesn't matter what type of fetish you have. We live in a world that fears anything out of the ordinary. Why do you think racism exists? Why are countries at war? At the root of both is the inability to accept something or someone that's different.

The human race is largely fear-based. We are raised to be mistrustful of others. We're protective of our belongings and contemptuous of older or younger generations. In general, we are most comfortable within rigid boundaries and borders. While we have the intelligence to be free, loving and open, we cling to what we know. The human race has been subjected to trauma from the moment we were evacuated from Eden. The repeated traumas of war, atrocities, and natural disasters have produced a species filled with deep-seated anxiety and abandonment issues.

We embrace steadfast rules, ideas and lifestyles because we crave safety. Look at young people. They work hard at "fitting in." They like to wear the same clothes, listen to the same music and be exactly like their peers. I even know of a group of teens who sport the same tattoo on the nape of their necks which says "to be different" in Chinese characters. If that's not being the same, I don't know what is! "Fitting in" is a quality that's valued. If someone stands out, they are subjected to ridicule and bullying. We're comfortable being cookie-cutter reproductions of each other.

Anything that's different is doomed to ridicule. Sex is especially uncomfortable because it's something private and primal. Most threatening of all, sex creates feelings of vulnerability. That's because in sexual moments we are out of control, especially during orgasm. Therefore, sex is inherently threatening. It brings us out of our comfort zone.

Society has attempted to keep itself under control by creating rules and regulations about when, how and with whom to have sex. Over the years, there have been deviations like homosexuality, bisexuality and lesbianism. But they are never truly embraced, only mildly tolerated. This civilization wants us to all fit into a mold. When we deviate, we are considered deviant. In this mode of thought, when you have a fetish, you see yourself as defective.

No wonder then, that you, as a fetishist, have so many issues. You're the guy who gets aroused by something out of the norm. You've known it since you were little. How awful you must have felt to make the connection. You immediately fled into fear. Fear of being found out. Fear of being an outcast. And the fear that you're doomed. This is because being different equals danger. See how it all connects?

You are aroused by something that's unconventional. Period. It doesn't even matter what it is. The fact that you're different triggers shame. That's why the foot fetishist interprets his fetish the same way as you do. Trust me, he thinks that his fetish is as outrageous as anybody else's. That's why fetish content isn't really relevant; all fetishists think they're bizarre. Once again, it goes back to your feelings about being a fetishist or getting aroused by something you perceive as odd. Remember this interpretation comes from you and your thinking!

Less-Common Fetishes

Let's take a moment to acknowledge you, the man with a fetish that is a bit more "out there." You've turned to this chapter because you feel as though your fetish is a little more intricate, unusual or uncommon. You're the person who will say to me:

> *"It's bad enough I have fetish, but it's even worse because my fetish is so _____."*

In the blank, fill in the word you'd use to describe your fetish.

Some of you might have used words like "abnormal," "kooky" or "crazy." It's strange and offbeat. People might hear about your fetish and react incredulously. "What!?" "How could that possibly turn you on?" Yet it does. You probably have trouble believing it yourself. Yet, it's the case.

You may have used words such as "disgusting," "distasteful," or "off-putting." Not all fetishes are pretty or neat. Despite your intellectual sensibilities your primal turn-on is just plain graphic. In truth, an erect penis has no conscience. It wants what it wants. The fantasy won't go away. You might not be able to fully act upon it but you have to admit, it's sure fun to think about. And you can. Wouldn't it be nice to have the thoughts minus the negative editorializing?

Name Dropping - An Honorable Mention of Some Fetishes Considered Uncommon

Less-common fetishes include anything that's highly distinctive, complex or simply unorthodox. Luckily, with the advent of the Internet, you may actually be able to Google your fetish and find that you aren't alone. This will feel shocking but validating.

Those of you who do a search and come up empty, remember to be careful of how you think. If you call yourself a name such as "freak," remember that you are both placing unfair labels upon yourself as well as thinking in terms of black and white. You are much more than the name you call yourself!

And does that term really describe you fully? I doubt it. Instead, think of the truth. You must be highly creative to have a fetish that is uniquely yours. I bet you are an interesting guy who has a good deal to share with the world. Remember that you can think however you choose to think, but in the end, you have this fetish. You didn't choose it; it chose you. Change your perception and you will change the way you feel.

Offbeat Fetish Role Call

In no apparent order is my collection of offbeat fetishes, which include:

The Old Pie in the Face

It's hard to imagine that anyone would enjoy having a pie thrown in their face. Yet, I personally know one man who has been very vocal about his penchant for whipped cream smashed in his kisser...publicly. And there are others like him. The odd part is that these fetishists are sexually aroused by something that most would find funny, assaultive or annoying.

If pie-tossing is you thing, ask yourself what type of pie you like tossed at you? Something creamy or gooey? Is it whipped cream that gets you going or fruit filling? Is it the humiliation aspect or the messy aspect? These are important questions to ask.

Furries and Plushies

Furries is a fetish that's confusing because the costuming is certainly not traditionally sexy to most people. Yet, if you think about it, the fetish actually makes sense—getting erotically charged by cute, furry, animal characters. People age 40 and younger grew up having contact with Animatronic figures and larger-than-life characters in amusement parks. Their first physical contact with any being outside of their parents just might have been with Big Bird or Cookie Monster. Something emotionally-charged happened in that moment and voila, a furry is born!

If you're a furry, remember to identify exactly what you like about the fetish. What's your character? How do you relate to other characters? What are your verbal cues? What do you imagine doing while dressed? Is your role passive or aggressive?

The furries fetish is sometimes referred to as a plushies fetish, although some purists contend that there are profound differences. Although plushies can focus more on smaller, stuffed or "plush" animals, I feel that for our purposes, the basis of the fetishes are essentially the same, so I group them together.

Casting

Casting is another fetish that appears to be nonsexual but if this is your fetish, you love the idea of wearing a cast. This can range from wearing a sling on your arm to a full body cast of plaster of Paris. You might enjoy wearing a neck brace as well. There is a Dominant/submissive component to this fetish since there can be a top or a bottom component. Some like to apply the cast; others like to wear it.

During your Identification Process, you will have to decide if you are a top, bottom or switch when it comes to casting.

You will also have to ask yourself: Is casting an activity you like to do alone or with another person? What aspects are essential? Do you like going out in public to get attention or would you rather be home alone?

Casting is actually considered to be a "cousin" to bondage. Especially if you get a charge from feeling helpless. It's an uncommon fetish but as it turns out, not as uncommon as I originally thought. The first time I ever heard of it was when a patient mentioned that they met their partner on a casting site. I'd assumed they were in the entertainment business. Boy, was I wrong. But I was very open to being educated about the casting fetish and not only discovered that there were indeed websites dedicated to it but a healthy casting community in full swing.

Poppers

People known as "poppers" are turned on by balloon-popping. That can make for an unusual party experience! There's most likely a direction correlation with the fear of hearing a balloon pop when you were a kid. It's another charged experienced that in some way, became sexualized.

If you're a popper, identify exactly what kind of balloons you like to see popped. Colors? Textures? Do you want to be the one doing the popping or do you want to watch your significant other do it? What aspect of popping turns you on—the act of popping, the sound or the balloon breaking?

Many readers who don't have this fetish, would think it's relatively easy to enact. However, many poppers will experience the negativity described in Chapter 18. Your woman might feel as though you like the balloon more than you like her. Your challenge is getting her to understand that you want to integrate her into the fetish by having her involved. It's not so much the balloon but her popping the balloon.

Castration

Here's a fetish/fantasy that you'd only be able to do once! I'm talking about castration. Clearly, this is only a fantasy but the fetish revolves around your arousal about the thought of being turned into a eunuch. Again, this is a very intricate fetish.

Your Identification Process would need to hone in on exactly what castration means to you. Is it about the ultimate sacrifice? Submitting to a dominant female in an extreme way? Wanting to be sexless? Is it connected to humiliation?

There are a small group of people who actually do succumb to the castration fantasy. Some do it to end hypersexual feelings. Others do it because they don't feel like they identify with being male or female. They call themselves eunuchs. It's a very difficult, extreme choice to make and in most cases, best left to fantasy.

Cosplay

Many young people are very into cosplay, which entails dressing in intricate costumes with or without a partner. The costumes are based on characters from specific movies, comic books or video games. While cosplay is not a fetish per se, these days there may be an undercurrent of sexual interaction. Some of the costumes are very sexually revealing. Some people also use cosplay as a form of cross-dressing. This is called "gender bending" because a character who would generally be female might be played by a male or vice versa. Sailor Moon, a Japanese manga character, is a favorite of men who like to gender bend with their cosplay. Role-playing is also something enjoyed by cosplayers.

Golden Showers, Brown Showers, Roman Showers and Farting

The above mentioned fetishes are all related. I group them together because all four involve "taboo" bodily functions. If you like golden showers, brown showers, Roman showers and farting, it means that you have a fetish for bodily waste, be it urine, feces, vomit or gas, respectively. You know that this fetish is definitely something difficult to explain. Each of them is less common than other fetishes, yet that's what turns you on. Which is fine and dandy.

Your Identification Process will include the context of the fetish which arouses you. Ask yourself what aspect of the fetish turns you on: Is it the waste product? Is it being forced? Is it being under the control of a Dominant? Is this part of a D/s exchange? Do you actually want to experience your fetish or would you prefer just being threatened with it? These are all key questions to ponder.

Totally Taboo Fetishes

This book is a judgment-free zone. No fetish is too unusual or too "freaky," unless it's illegal. Things like pedophilia aren't tolerated; and they aren't fetishes, but disorders. It is illegal and morally wrong to have sex with a person under the age of 18.

Also frowned upon are fetishes that cross the law in other ways. Case in point, the much publicized fetish of Jordan D. Haskins, the 24-year-old GOP candidate for Michigan's legislature. It seems that Haskins has a long, criminal history which dates back to age 15 for trespassing and vehicle break-ins. When confronted with his criminal record, Haskins confessed that he took pleasure in "cranking," a fetish which involves disconnecting a car's ignition wires and masturbating while restarting the car engine.

Cranking is similar to flashing or exposing oneself to someone who is unsuspecting or unknowing. Yes, you could say they are fetishes too but the difference between these illegal fetishes and the ones that I'm covering in this book is very simple. When it comes to doing anything that is against someone's will, it puts another human being in danger. If you suffer from this, I do urge you to get help. I realize it's difficult because therapists have a "duty to report" anything that is considered a sexual crime. I hate this aspect of the law because it might be preventing you from learning how to get your inclinations under control.

I suggest that you go to an anonymous 12-step program and start to listen at the meetings. You are not under any obligation to speak or confess anything about your past. I also urge you to work on your anxiety, be forgiving of yourself and learn how to manage whatever you're doing. Remember your victims. They might be traumatized by your acts and I know you don't want to hurt anyone.

I want to make it clear that the kind of fetishes I'm talking about in this book are legal and consensual. They are not to be confused with things like cranking or flashing, which could be fetishist but are against the law if not done with another person's consent. The distinction must be made because the general public lumps them all together. Please realize that there is a huge difference between a fetish that is practiced alone or with a consenting adult and a fetish that is used to scare, shock or intimidate people.

The Solution

The problem with many unusual fetishes is that they are difficult to enact. That's why you feel frustrated and envious of those who have fetishes that are easier to bring to life. In contrast, you have fantasy-based fetishes. Anyone who has a castration fantasy knows that he probably wouldn't want to do it in reality. But it's exciting to think about. Likewise, many men (especially submissives) like the idea of wearing chastity belts. They think they'll like it—until someone locks them into one! At that moment, the erection will turn flaccid and he just wants out!

The common theme for identified unusual fetishes is the shock value. And this is where I'll find some truth in your skepticism. These fetishes are more difficult to explain than some of the more common fetishes. These fetishes seemingly fall from the realm of what we conceive to be sexual contact. How in the world does popping a balloon or throwing a pie in someone's face translate into romantic sex? How is it possible to equate sexuality with casting? Bodily fluids like vomit? It seems impossible to connect the dots.

Yet, it is indeed possible because it's a fetish. This is where your uncommon fetish holds the same challenge as all the rest. You must be knowledgeable and comfortable with your fetish in order to explain it to another person. True, your fetish might be "out there" but your ability to communicate can make fetish fulfillment possible. You just need to do the back-office work!

The Uncommon Fetish Case Studies

I've personally worked with several men who have pretty uncommon fetishes. Together, we came up with workable solutions, which I'd like to share with you here.

Uncommon Fetish Case Study # 1 - Amazon Women

Amir likes women who are of Amazonian proportions. He likes to envision them overpowering him by wrestling. He fantasizes about a muscular seven foot tall giantess who overtakes him to the point of no return—smothering him between her massive thighs. Amir came to me because he felt sad. In essence, he said that he wanted a woman that doesn't exist, a woman who only lives in Fantasyland.

Uncommon Fetish Case Study # 2 - The Superheroine

Peter had a similar fantasy to Amir's. He liked the idea of women who were based on strong, invincible Superhero characters. Someone who had the power to make him shrink so small that she'd be able to put him in her pocket and take him with her wherever she went. Again, pretty impossible, but still, it aroused Peter to no end.

Uncommon Fetish Case Study # 3 – Cooked and Eaten

Phillip must have watched too many Bugs Bunny cartoons when he was little because he had a fantasy of being cooked in a hot cauldron of water. He then wanted to be trussed up and eaten like a chicken. Good fantasy, but it's not reality-based. How could this possibly happen in real life?

Uncommon Fetish Case Study # 4 – Blinded by Love

Nick is excited by the idea of being blinded by a dominant female. "I'll gouge out your eyeballs" is a phrase he loved to hear. Though this fantasy is unusual, it actually can be enacted because Nick likes the verbiage more than the act. His challenge was to find a woman who was willing to whisper this phrase instead of sweet nothings like "I love you" during sex. As a result, Nick was driven to find a woman who was as enthusiastic about his fetish as he was.

How these Uncommon Case Studies (and Your Unusual Fetish) Can Be Enacted

It's true that some fetishes are impossible to bring to fruition. While huge women may exist, will that super-tall Amazon translate into a life partner for you? Sadly, it isn't likely.

Superheroes simply don't exit. Plus, Phillip and Nick have such distinctive tastes that there are no websites fully devoted to their specific desires. (Yet.) In lieu of starting their own fetish websites, how can they share their fantasies?

Solution: Storytelling

Storytelling sounds so simple, but it works. Incredibly well. And it's so easy…and best of all, it's free! Storytelling has been mentioned previously as a means to bring a reluctant partner into your fetish world. This storytelling option also worked for Amir, Peter, Phillip and Nick. It even worked for a friend of mine, who had no interest in submitting to her husband's anal sex fantasies (her hemorrhoids were a big deterrent!) but the mere mention of backdoor romance and a detailed description of the act during standard vaginal sex sent her hubby over the edge.

To successfully carry out storytelling, you have to complete the outlined tasks designed for all fetishes. Educate yourself about your fetish. Identify all aspects of your individual fetish, including all the components necessary to bring it to life. You then have to brush up on your communication skills in order to clearly articulate your wishes to your partner.

If you have an unusual fetish that can't be enacted real time, storytelling is a viable option. This is assuming you have clearly communicated your fetish needs and your lady is ready to participate.

Storytelling simply gives the two of you an opportunity to share in your fetish together. Your partner will actually bring your fetish to life by talking about it. That way, you hear her voice while imagining your most intimate, secret longings. This is real intimacy that can be enjoyed by a fetishist and his wife. It works.

Happy Endings

Through some creative storytelling, Amir's partner can truly say that she's grown to be seven feet tall.

So can Peter's wife. She can then describe all the ways she would overtake him, according to Peter's explicit instructions, which include specific verbiage and catch phrases that get him going.

Phillip's girlfriend will tell him that she's going to cook him in a cauldron of boiling water and turn him into a delicious stew, which he loves to no end.

Nick's wife has it the easiest She can go into exquisite detail about blinding him. She will also incorporate the sentence, "I'm going to gouge out your eyeballs" over and over again until he quivers in a shattering climax. And hopefully, she does too, just knowing how much she's just aroused her man.

During the storytelling, you will pleasure yourself and orgasm from her words. She can also take matters into hand as she spins her fetish yarns. Or you can simply use the stories as foreplay. It's a choice to be made by you and your partner.

Please remember that these stories can be saved for special occasions. Your wife will probably be happy to do this sometimes. Just like some people use sexy lingerie as an occasional treat, it's not always on the menu. However, always take into consideration that she's your partner through all of this and it's also important to take into consideration her feelings and wishes. I'm confident that with a lot of discussion and a healthy portion of thoughtfulness, your story will have a happy ending, too.

In Summary

While it's true that some fetishes may seem more challenging than others, the work required is always the same:

1) Learn about your fetish;
2) Identify what you enjoy; and
3) Don't rule out the possibility that your partner will want to join in with you no matter how outrageous your fantasy appears.

Never forget that success is all about your confidence and your attitude.

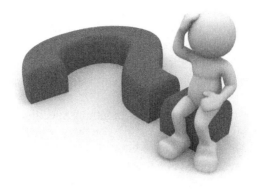

Chapter 16 - Should You Share Your Fetish with Your Partner?

You have a fetish that is uniquely yours. At this point, you have come to a place of understanding and acceptance. You have done your due diligence and have made a thorough identification of what your fetish entails. This is for your own self-knowledge. And, of course, it will be the blueprint to use for any kind of real-time fantasy fulfillment.

You realize that it's not so much about *why* you have a fetish as much as it's about the fact that you do have a fetish. You realize that your sexual fetish is strong, powerful and will never go away. With that knowledge, you have a choice. You can beat yourself up and think you're weird, perverse or sick. Or you can choose to tell yourself that you have something that's quirky, off-the-beaten-track and unique.

You know that your worth is not based on the fact that you happen to have a sexual fetish. It's merely a small part of who you are. The fact that you have a sexual fetish just means that you're turned on by something out of the norm. That's it. Big deal. You're not a serial killer; you're just a guy who likes his sex served up a bit differently. What's so wrong about that?

As it turns out, sexuality is not as rigid as was once thought. People are aroused by all sorts of things. I sometimes compare it to the way people like different types of foods. Some like Thai, others like sushi, and still others like Ethiopian cuisine. None of them is better than the other or more "right." Some people love ethnic food and others find it repugnant. And it's the same with fetish.

Similarly, you happen to have something specific that gets you going. Consider yourself lucky. You have something that reliably turns you on, no matter what. This means you'll be feeling erotic, well past your sexual prime, as long as you allow yourself to think of your fetish.

No matter how much you might want to wish your fetish away, it's here to stay. The best course of action is to accept the fact that your fetish is but one small component of who you are. It doesn't have to define you as a human being. It doesn't have to make you an outcast. It also doesn't have to condemn you to a lifetime of masturbation or loneliness.

However, before you jump up and blurt out your fetish to your current partner, potential partner or the person sitting next to you on the bus, let's give this some real thought. Thoughtfulness is key to healthy fetish management.

To Tell or Not to Tell?

Now, we come to the big question—to tell or not to tell— which sparks many other questions:

- Should you, would you or does it make sense for you to share your fetish with another human being?
- Is it appropriate to divulge your fetish while dating? If so, when do you tell them?
- What about if you're already married? Is it advantageous or appropriate to bring up something you've been secretive about for years?
- What are the benefits of telling and when does it make more sense to keep your mouth shut and compartmentalize?

These are all very valid questions that plague many fetishists. A fetish is so complex, yet so present. If fetish is a part of you and you want to share all parts of you with your partner, then it seems to make perfect sense to share. Sharing is a no-brainer. Yet you find the risk of rejection overwhelmingly daunting.

Again, that's why self-acceptance and self-discussion is still the key. Don't even think about revealing your fetish until you are personally healed. You'll have to study your thought process and then work some more before you can discuss it another person.

Understanding how your thoughts affect your feelings and self-beliefs is challenging and takes dedication. It's like working out. You can go to the gym once and learn a few routines, but in order to build up muscle, you have to keep repeating these routines. Building up your self-esteem takes perseverance. However, it's essential in order for you to be able to express yourself correctly to your current partner or someone you're dating.

For now, let's assume you're feeling pretty good about yourself and your fetish. (That means this book has done its job!) In fact, you're feeling so comfortable that no one, not even the person you love most in this world, will be able to shatter your self-image. You understand that you're a good person. You contribute to society and are generous to those you love. You are not disordered. You only engage in your fetish with consenting adults. And you're well-intentioned about your desire to divulge.

What do I mean by "well-intentioned?" Agreed, it's a very subjective phrase. But generally speaking, one who is well-intentioned wants to do what is best for the situation at hand without personal gain. The well-intentioned fetishist wants to share or not share based upon the dynamic of an existing relationship.

To be truly well-intentioned, you must honestly evaluate your own relationship and do what's best for both you and your partner. Your relationship may change positively, negatively or even implode. Remember that old proverb, "The road to hell is paved with good intentions"? Even the best-intentioned acts can backfire, so you need to prepare as best you can to ensure it goes as well as it can.

Now, it's all up to you. Take a deep breath and consider…

Reasons Not to Tell

Yes, even the well-intentioned person might not want to tell their partner about their fetish. Remember, we are defining "well-intentioned" as one who is looking at the whole picture and wanting to do what is best for everyone involved. The well-intentioned person makes a decision for the good of all.

Some of you might be discovering your fetish later on in life. You might be married for decades and only now are allowing yourself the luxury of acknowledging that you have sexual predilections considered by most people to be "out of the norm." Is it fair for you to spring this on your wife of 10, 20, or 30 years? Is it a good idea to let it be known that you have been keeping a big sexual fantasy under wraps?

Generally-speaking, in a case where you are married for decades, it's probably best to keep your fetish to yourself. You have survived this long and you can survive some more. The difference is that now you have more of an understanding about your fetish so you can allow yourself to think about it at the moment of orgasm without feeling guilty or creepy. Your fetish belongs to you and it is what it is. No shame. No remorse

You know your partner. How does she react to change? To things out of the ordinary? Is your fetish something she would embrace or would you be causing a wedge in your relationship? Though I wish I could be more optimistic about having you tell a long-term partner, my experience with counseling fetishists indicates that springing something big on your partner usually doesn't work.

Instead, let me suggest that you find some creative ways to get your wants met indirectly. For example, if you like the idea of being submissive, you can "serve" her by placing more emphasis on her climax. Do sweet things for her like draw her a bath, massage her and service her to orgasm. Do it with a submissive mindset. She'll never know the difference, it's not harmful in any way, and she'll love the attention!

If you have a fetish for a specific body part, you can indulge in it without saying anything. So, if you're a foot fetishist, rub her feet and sneak in a few kisses. If you are a hair fetishist, you can comb her hair spontaneously. If you like long fingernails treat her to a trip to the manicurist's. And if you like particular clothing, buy it for her. Do your best not to act too eager about having her try them on. Just act casual. Tell her you think she'd look hot in the pantyhose, panties or boots, and spur her forward with compliments. Flattery and gifts are things few can resist.

Remember to reassure your lady that these outfits were bought because you want her to wear the clothing—and know she'll look fabulous in it. This is a very important detail. Fetishists often blow it because they come on too strong or too eager. This is completely understandable but never forget that women are very cerebral. They'll notice anything out of the ordinary and question your motive.

Women worry about being objectified in terms of a fetish. They worry that you love the article of fetish more than you love them. Remember, you have chosen not to tell, so it's important not to blow your cover. Downplay your desires. Simply tell her that you were thinking about the way she'd look in the leather, panties, pantyhose, etc. Leave it at that and don't pressure her. If she doesn't take the initiative to put it on, remind her at a time when you're both feeling relaxed. Be flirtatious. You'll usually get good results.

Honestly, she doesn't have to know everything about you or the fact that you have a fetish. I'm sure there are private things about herself that she doesn't share with you. We all have secret compartments within ourselves. You're not being dishonest with her, though. But rather, you're thinking of a way to involve her in your fetish without igniting a major fire. Your fetish is the key to your arousal. You want to be excited and you'd prefer to be excited by your partner. Does that make you such a bad guy? I think not, and hope you agree.

Of course, the idea would be for your partner to be aware of your sexual triggers so you can interact together mindfully. This would be the ideal but sometimes it's not always possible. If that's the case with you, think about ways to covertly bring your fetish into the bedroom. And who knows, unconsciously she just might put two and two together and make the connection on her own. If she's having fun and having a good time with you, she just might get the idea. That would be fantastic, wouldn't it?

Almost every long-term relationship needs a little spicing up. So what if yours requires props, special clothing or contact with body parts not ordinarily associated with traditional sex? Really...so what?

Any Other Reasons Not to Tell?

Some fetishists decide not to reveal their cravings by choice. You want to keep your fantasy a fantasy. You might prefer to read stories, watch DVDs or fantasize in a clandestine setting. But in no way do you want to share. Your fetish is your own private masturbatory material. Your fetish is a solitary activity by choice. And as such, it must be managed and controlled along those lines.

If that's how you feel, it might be helpful to think of your fetish as a hobby, something you partake in by yourself. You can enjoy the hobby as a pleasurable pastime but you still need to work, pay bills and live life. Your hobby cannot over take your relationship and has to take a back seat to everything else in your life. Although you allow space for the hobby activity, it can't interfere with other aspects of your existence.

Spouses often have no interest in their partner's hobby, although they do know of their husband's interests. Building birdhouses, going kayaking—or in your case, cross-dressing— holds no interest for them whatsoever. But they're fine with their partner doing it.

However, a fetish is a bit different than baking bread or making model airplanes. If you choose to keep your fetish a secret, you are choosing to withhold an important element of your sexuality from your partner. Sexual relations are something life-partners vow to share with each other. Keeping your fetish private is your choice to make as long as it doesn't interfere with the overall quality of your relationship. This means you don't get to spend hours alone at your computer. Instead, you get to spend time together. You get to interact and you get to maintain intimacy with your wife.

Conversely, some fetishists believe that their offbeat predilections get in the way of existing or potential relationships. I say: Only if you let it. A number off my professional colleagues disagree. They'll tell you that you can't focus on the fetish at the expense of your wife. They'll warn you that watching fetish pornography will desensitize your desire for sex. In short, they don't understand or acknowledge that having a fetish is a real necessity. If anything, the Internet has been a blessing for fetishists. Finally, you don't feel so alone. Finally, you don't feel like you're "the only one."

But like anything else, you have to be careful and indulge in your fetish the same as you'd indulge in any luxury. If you love to golf, you have to pick and choose your tee times. If you love to eat rich, fatty foods, you learn to eat them sparingly — and savor every bite. I know you get my point. Healthy balance is essential in everything we do.

Remember, it's your choice to keep your fetish for masturbatory pleasure alone. But it doesn't have to be your choice to isolate it from your present or potential partner.

You can't expunge a fetish. It is deeply ingrained. However, you can manage your fetish by giving yourself choice. You can choose to accept your fetish and choose when and whom to tell. Once you gain control of your ship, you can steer it toward health, happiness and intimate relationships. You can have a relationship and be a fetishist. Millions do. The key is making choices, thinking rationally and gaining control.

With that said, there are many good reasons to share your fetish. After all, it's only one part of you. It doesn't define you. But it is a part of who you are and definitely a huge component of your sexual makeup. Many self-accepting fetishists are adamant about telling, especially those who are single and dating.

Who Do You Tell?

I think the answer to this is pretty simple. The person/s you tell are those whom you are sexually intimate with. After all, would you tell your next-door neighbor that you love getting blow jobs? Would you tell your work colleagues your favorite sex positions? They fall under the category of TMI. And seriously, how much do you really divulge about your sexual preferences to casual acquaintances anyway? How truthful is your sex talk between buddies? If you have one special friend you confide in then, maybe you'd talk about your fetish with him or her. But ultimately, the person you talk sex with is the person you would share your fetish with.

Remember, at this point, we're referring to sharing information. We're not even discussing participation. Performing and enacting your fetish is a whole other topic. This section is simply about sharing something about yourself with someone whom you are currently or planning to be intimate with.

I always say that the right person is the one who will be open-minded and accepting. If she isn't and you aren't in a committed relationship, now is a good time to rethink that relationship, and possibly end it. Not because of the fetish itself but because if she isn't accepting of your sexual fantasies, then she might not be accepting of your other dreams. True, your fetish doesn't define you but it's a big part of your sexuality. It's important to choose your partners wisely. The "fetish test" is a good barometer to judge compatibility on many levels.

Talking about your fetish opens the gateway toward real intimacy and closeness. It allows you to be vulnerable. That's why I advocate telling someone whom you are considering for a long-term relationship. If you're heading in a direction of making a commitment, most fetishists agree that it's wise to divulge the fetish before making that final commitment.

Does this mean you tell them on the third or fourth date? That's a personal choice. Many fetishists who are dating do recommend talking about a fetish within the first couple of months. It's kind of like a screening process. Just consider it part of getting to know each other better and sharing.

Make sure you don't talk about your fetish like it's an infliction or disease; it's isn't. Don't address it as though it's shameful because it's not that either. However, do discuss it with the respect it deserves—you're sharing it with this special person because you want to allow yourself to be vulnerable and open about who you are with someone you think you'd like to get even closer with. It's a huge chunk of personal information and the very essence of you.

This is why I think telling a potential person about your fetish is so valuable and dear. In essence, you are giving her the key to absolute understanding about you and your sexuality. You are giving her the key that allows her to be the very best lover she can be. If she takes this key with an attitude of respect and gratitude, she's getting the most valuable information she could ever receive from you.

Your revelation is a gift and should be seen as such. It's not learning something off-putting but it's useful knowledge about what makes you tick. You're allowing her access to your vulnerability. Again, it's about her learning and seeing things from a different perspective.

Conversely, the woman who is scornful of your fetish is the woman you should eject from your life. Run, don't walk! She's not the woman for you or anyone else, for that matter. Her reaction demonstrates that she's selfish and narrow-minded. Your existence will be limiting with her as your life partner, and not just where your fetish is concerned; where everything is concerned.

Talking about your fetish is necessary, but it's only necessary with someone whom you care to be close with. Fetish couples are often closer than their straight counterparts. Once you talk to your woman about your fetish, the two of you will have the opportunity to consider the next step. Do you want to bring your fetish to life? And if so, how?

But please realize that even if the fetish is never enacted, the two of you will be closer and more intimate than ever. This is assuming she's okay with it, and willing to accept and acknowledge your fetish. If that's the case, you're in a good place and you're with the right woman. Secrets and secretive behaviors are gone. You don't have to sneak to the computer to visit sites devoted to your fetish. You don't have to hide your props and toys. You're free to be who you are: The nice guy who happens to have a quirky fetish.

Telling Your Partner

Disclosing your fetish is the optimal way to go. Optimal, but very, very challenging. And, of course, there are numerous factors to consider, like:

Are you in a new relationship?

Many fetishists are resolute in their quest to be with a person who will accept, understand and hopefully, participate in their fetish needs. If you're one of these people, then having "the fetish talk" is required within the first few months of the relationship. That's because you have decided that your fetish is a deal-breaker. If she's not willing to participate, then you aren't willing to continue your relationship.

As someone who's dating, you must be clear about your options, especially if you're dating with the hope of something long-term. If you want your fetish in your life and you want it with your partner, then you simply have to be with someone who's willing to participate. There's no way around this one. You know your options. Make a decision and stick to your goals. If you bring up the topic and she's closed, antagonistic or derogatory, get out. I don't care how hot she is or how much you think you love her. If you don't want to be secretive, sneaky or rejected, you absolutely have to get out. Now!

Are you in a long-term relationship?

Revealing a fetish in a long-term relationship is a more difficult decision. At this moment, you're feeling a sense of inner peace and acceptance about your fetish. You realize that it isn't so bad and that morally, intellectually and spiritually, there's nothing inherently wrong with having something eccentric that turns you on. You wish you had broached the subject with your significant other years ago, but alas and alack, you didn't.

Just don't beat yourself up over it because you weren't emotionally ready to share your fetish at the time. You were too shy and uncomfortable about it. You didn't have the knowledge or understanding that you possess today. You thought you could repress your arousals and hoped that your fetish thoughts would simply go away. I know because I have spoken to thousands of people just like you.

Don't be your own whipping boy. (Unless you're into self-flagellation!) Instead, give some serious thought to the pros and cons of broaching the subject with your partner.

It might help you organize your feelings if you actually draw a line down the middle of a piece of paper. On the left-hand column, list how it will help your relationship to disclose your fetish after all these years. On the right-hand column, list how disclosure will hurt your relationship. Only you can decide which column carries the most weight. Sometimes it helps seeing your choices written down in black-and-white. Notice that I included the word "relationship" in your pros and cons list. This is a relationship decision because it affects the two of you. Don't be selfish about it, just be honest.

I also want you to be attentive to where you're at in your relationship. Many choose to disclose their fetish after a long period of time, say, after the kids are grown. Others choose to disclose because they're unhappy with their partner and use their fetish as leverage for ending the relationship.

Please be thoughtful and create your pros and cons list in the spirit of making an improvement in your life. If you want to leave your long-term relationship, end it because other things aren't going well. Don't use your fetish as an excuse. It won't work out well for you or your partner.

As much as the notion of revelation frightens you, it can also help strengthen your bond. I know that's difficult to believe but it's true. More often than not, fetishists are aching to "spill the beans" because they're tired of keeping a secret. They feel it's incredibly cathartic to get their fetish off their chest, and their partner is grateful they were secure enough in their relationship to share this most personal piece of themselves.

But again, only disclose if your significant other will benefit from knowing the most private aspect of your being. She can benefit because now she has a better of understanding of what makes you "you." Telling her divulges the secret to your sexuality. She now has the magic recipe of how to be your best lover. If she is an open-minded person and you honestly believe it will help the relationship, then yes, go ahead and tell her. It will feel good to get that skeleton out of your closet—especially when you see it wasn't so scary in the first place. And so many things looks frightening in the dark, don't they?

Maybe your partner has had an inkling about your fetish all along. If that's the case, then you might want to go ahead and disclose. You probably feel you have nothing to lose.

But I also want to emphasize that revealing your fetish isn't fool-proof. You can lose your relationship. If you think she has an idea about your fetish and has been snooping into your online history, then you have no choice but to tell her. However, be careful about how you do this. Remember to be positive in both the language you use and your general attitude. A good way to start might be to simply tell her the truth when she "outs" you. 'What a relief!' you can begin. 'I've been dying to tell you for years but I just didn't know how.'

Another benefit on the plus side of the column might be about spicing things up in the bedroom. Fetish play accomplishes exactly that. Remember, it's play. Amusement...recreation...relaxation. It's a wonderful blessing to allow ourselves the luxury of play, even into our twilight years. Most of the time, fetish play does not necessitate use of our genital area. Therefore, it's perfect for the menopausal woman who might be experiencing symptoms of vaginal dryness or lack of sexual desire. She can dress in an empowering dominant outfit, use sex toys, play implements, and doesn't have to think twice about lubrication.

Fetish play can also be the perfect antidote for those who have trouble performing in the conventional way. Fetish participation can potentially add a wonderful new line of communication between you and your partner. Fetish lends itself to talking, visiting alternative websites together and going on shopping sprees to get supplies. Fetish is definitely fun! It all has to do with attitude.

But a revelation about fetish interest deep into a long-term relationship can also hurt when a long-standing partner feels betrayed. "Why didn't you tell me before?," they might ask. "How could you have kept such a big secret from me?" Yes, there may be a barrage of questions following your revelation, so be prepared to answer them honestly and openly. If you keep a cool head and provide heartfelt, real, rational answers, the end result still might be positive. You just have to be patient and weather the storm of her very valid emotions.

Of course, her reaction might also be antagonistic. She could call you a pervert or a freak and accuse you of being a sex addict. This is exactly why you didn't tell her in the first place. However, at this point you have adapted an attitude of positive, unconditional self-compassion. Her words will bounce off your brain like a brand new Super Ball. You'll be deaf to her complaints. They won't get to you. Their negativity will not penetrate you.

A negative response will be the worst your fetish revelation gets. Only you can decide if the possible benefits outweigh the potential detriments. Telling your long-term partner about your fetish is tricky and risky. Ultimately, the choice is yours: to tell or not to tell. Be sensitive to what's best for your relationship.

In Summary

Discussing your fetish is in the same category as any kind of self-disclosure. The more you get to know someone, the closer you will allow them to get. When dating, you first want to know if your partner will be receptive to your fetish. Use common sense. Even in traditional relationships, sexuality becomes more open and more intimate as the relationship progresses.

But your fetish can also be a deal-breaker if you want a long-term relationship which includes fetish. Be hip to this in your communication. Don't wait too long to tell a partner. Get "the fetish talk" out in the open and over with when you know there could be real potential in the relationship.

Talking to your long-term mate has its benefits and disadvantages. Weigh them carefully before moving ahead with revealing your fetish.

Don't forget that fetish is all about intimacy and trust. The closer you get, the more you'll feel comfortable in disclosing. Your Identification Process contains all the details of your fetish. If you decide to bring the fetish to life, you will divulge as much or as little as you deem correct. At this point, you know the difference between needs and wants. Hopefully, in the beginning, you'll realize that a little goes a long way.

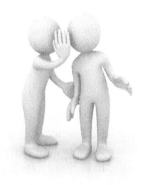

Chapter 17 – Communication: How to Tell Her

Communication. This is a word which many people use, yet most of us don't really know the true meaning of. What does communication entail? According to the Merriam-Webster Online Dictionary, communication is "the act or process of using words, sounds, signs, or behaviors to express or exchange information or to express your ideas, thoughts, feelings, etc., to someone else." Sounds easy enough, doesn't it?

As human beings, we're communicating with each other all the time. Even when we think we aren't. That's because our body language, facial expressions and the way we carry ourselves give off signals. It's often easy to figure out strong emotions others are experiencing. We observe telltale gestures like shaking legs, rocking or the wringing of hands. These movements indicate nervousness. We can also read people's emotions by their facial expressions. Or even by hearing sounds such as sighing, nervous laugher or clearing of the throat.

We all know how to communicate to some degree. The problem is making sure our listener understands the message. Our present challenge is to communicate about fetish. Congratulations, you've decided to tell another human being about your quirk. This person might be a professional, but hopefully it will be your spouse or partner. While most of this chapter will geared toward individuals who are telling their spouse or significant other, I do want to make an important point about disclosing your fetish to a professional.

Communicating to a Professional

Proper communication, even to a professional fantasy worker, is vital. The more you tell, the better she will be able to bring your fantasy to life. But no one is a mind reader, even a pro, and no two fetishists are alike. Some fetish requirements are yours and yours alone. That's why your Identification Processed required you to disclose every detail, no matter how seemingly small. These details are important for you and your unique fantasy. If something is missing or not addressed, your fetish scene will not be totally fulfilling.

Use your Identification List as a blueprint. Share your most important requirements, including props, costuming and verbiage. Because she is experienced in fetish fulfillment, the person you hired will be able to take it from there. Remember, you are paying for a service and this gives you the right to get the experience you want. If you're buying a household appliance like a coffee maker, you want to make sure you're getting one that fits you, correct? Paying for a fetish fantasy experience is not so different.

Before your session starts, you should take the lead and come well-prepared to communicate your desires. Then you can relax and get into fetish mode while playing.

Communicating with Your Spouse

When couples go for counseling, communication is always the topic most discussed. It turns out that we each have difficulties expressing ourselves, being heard and understanding when to listen. Men have a tendency to be "fixers." But making things all better may not necessarily be what women want. Women tend to have a desire to be listened to, whether the problem actually gets fixed or not.

Likewise, men have a desire for appreciation. Women often forget to acknowledge the nice things their husbands do for them. Couples counseling highlights the things we miss and gives us the opportunities to express ourselves more effectively.

Many of the techniques employed in relationship counseling are the very same ones you will use when talking to your spouse about your fetish. Empathy, self-expression and listening are the key skills you must to learn.

Understand that most of your spouses are unfamiliar with fetish. Along with that understanding, you'll have to remember the tools that helped you come to a place of self-acknowledgement. Remember, you've been struggling with fetish most of your life. Up until this point, it's the secret you planned to take to your grave. Through education, self-exploration and rational thinking, you've finally arrived at self-acceptance. Your challenge now is to help your partner get to the same place. It will take patience on your part but I'm confident you can do it. You've come this far!

I know you'll want to dive right in. I know you'll want to tell her everything all at once and expect her to eagerly participate. While you can wish for that, you must be mindful of the myriad of emotions she's experiencing. Remember that you gave yourself a good chunk of time to be at peace with your fetish. It's probably taken you years to be at peace with your fetish. Your spouse deserves the gift of time as well. A little will go a long way. Utilize my step-by-step guideline that includes basic communication skills. I can't make guarantees but I'm very hopeful. At the very least, it gives you a fighting chance.

Basic Communication Skills: Step-by-Step

I've compiled a list of some solid communication skills you'll find extremely useful in telling your partner about your fetish. But they'll also come in handy for other important life-changing conversations.

Empathy

Before you make your approach, put yourself in your partner's shoes. Imagine how she'll feel about learning the news about your having a fetish. She might think it's great, weird or strange.

Acknowledging her feelings before you even start is a good place to begin. Continuous empathy throughout your conversations will allow her to feel okay with her feelings. You'll simply be acknowledging how she's feeling.

A word to the wise: Never dispute a feeling. "Don't be angry at me" and "You shouldn't feel bad about this" are the kinds of sentences you don't want to use. After all, you don't want to tell her how she should and shouldn't feel any more than you'd want her to tell you that you should or shouldn't have a fetish.

Acknowledge her emotions with empathetic statements like, "This must be shocking for you to hear" or "I can't even imagine what you're feeling right now." Notice the difference. When using empathy, you allow her the space to feel whatever she feels.

Every human being is entitled to feel. It doesn't mean their feelings are necessarily fact, just that they're valid and should be acknowledged. And that's where you'll eventually move—from initial, knee-jerk reactions to more rational thinking. However, it's very important to allow her the time and space to feel and express.

Listening

Another way to show empathy and mindfulness is to listen to her and make sure you're hearing her correctly. Sure, you can guess how she's feeling but you also want to make sure you're getting the message she means to convey. To accomplish this, it's fine to actually repeat or paraphrase what she says. "In other words, you say you're feeling betrayed right now because I misrepresented myself to you," you could offer. Or "I'm hearing you say that you feel shocked because you don't think you know me anymore."

Basic listening allows the speaker to be heard correctly. These communications will undoubtedly produce feelings of anxiety in you as well as in your partner. After all, you never really shared something like this with her before. It's very natural for you to feel fearful and anxious. Often, when we're nervous, we retreat into our own heads. As a result, we miss out on what someone is saying.

By going into your own head, I mean that you're busy worrying about how she's reacting to your fetish instead of listening to her actually reacting to your fetish. This is why I want to caution you about zoning out. Instead, focus in on her. Make sure you understand exactly what she's saying. You can literally paraphrase what she says and then ask if you heard her correctly. Focusing in on her words and staying in the moment will also ease your own inner tensions. Maintaining eye contact is extremely helpful. Look at her while you're talking to her.

Find Truth in What She's Saying

Your natural reaction would be to go on the defensive. Your partner might express a great deal of negativity to you in the beginning. Rather than defend yourself, I would like you to find something in what she says that is the truth. If she calls you a name like weirdo, pervert or sex addict, simply agree in the following way:

> *"Yes, I guess I am a pervert. My fetish is certainly something that most people find strange and off-putting. I used to feel that way myself. But lately, I've come to understand exactly what my fetish means to me. I'd like to share what I've learned with you when you're ready."*

It works to find truth in whatever someone says to you, no matter how hurtful. After all, she's only using a label. By using the same word in a more rational fashion, you don't have to defend yourself and drive her further away. You simply agree, understand where she's coming from and self-disclose in order to further the discussion.

At this point, you've crossed an important threshold in breaking the news to her about your fetish. This discussion isn't necessarily a one-time talk but it's definitely a starting point. Basically, you're disclosing new information about yourself. Not only new, but very significant information. Allow her time to express herself as well as process the idea of fetish on her own. This is a lot to take in all at once. Remind yourself to be patient, kind and empathetic in your speech.

Don't get discouraged if her initial reaction leans toward the negative. This isn't really about you. Her inner dialogue will contain many anxious thoughts about your relationship. Most women go into a state of panic when hearing big news like discovering their partner's fetish. They jump to conclusions and spin worst case scenarios. "Aren't I enough for him?," " Will he leave me for someone else who has a fetish too?," "What if I can't handle this?" and "Is this the end of our marriage?" are many very valid fears that may be going through her head.

She might also be angry that you've withheld something big from her for a long time. As a result, she might feel betrayed and hurt. Give her time to absorb the information. Once she works through her own feelings, she'll be able to hear more about what you have to say. Just take a deep breath and be patient and loving with her.

Be Forthright and Confident

It's no secret that women like confident men. No matter how degrading, embarrassing or off-the-wall your fetish might seem, your presentation of it will make all the difference. Don't be apologetic. Speak from your heart in first person sentences. This is about you and your fetish, not her. That means you should steer away from saying things like, "You're so close-minded about sex," "You never want to talk about sex" or "You're so prudish when it comes to sex."

I suggest you begin your sentences with "I" statements. Things like: "I have something out of the ordinary that arouses me," "I've had to come to terms with my fetish and I don't believe it's going away" and "I want to incorporate this into our lives in a way that will be fun and healthy for the both of us."

Take Responsibility

Don't be accusatory. Avoid pointing the finger in her direction. While there may be truth in the fact that you hid your fetish because deep down you knew she'd be resistant, now is not the time to express your frustration. Do your best to stay on task. Ask yourself what you want in the long run. Remember your goal. You have made the decision to share your fetish with your wife. You don't want to live in secret any longer.

Many of you will be satisfied with gaining your partner's acceptance. Some of you may be hoping she'll eventually join in and play. Whatever you crave, stay focused on the big picture.

Remember, this isn't about settling the score. It's about getting her on your team—and scoring that game-winning goal together.

Not only do I want you to take responsibility; I'm asking you to take responsibility without apology. This means owning up to the fact that you did indeed hide your fetish from her. Speak from your heart and tell her why using by "I" statements. Sentences like: "I chose not to tell you based on my own feelings of fear and shame. I'm having trouble living with this now. But I've done a great deal of research to help myself accept this and I want to let you know what I've discovered."

If she's angry, allow her to have the feeling of anger. Don't defend yourself. She has every right to feel the way she does. She needs to vent. It's part of the process. Eventually, the important thing to deal with is the here and now, and you'll have a chance to do just that once she has had time to assimilate what you've just told her.

A good way to visualize your fetish is to see it as an ingredient sitting on your kitchen counter which is a necessary part of creating a balanced meal. It's important to focus on the idea of making a dinner which is satisfying to you both. Remind her that it's always better to savor a meal together.

Reframe

Another important element of communication is reframing. Therapists use this all the time. Instead of dwelling on the negatives, be more realistic in your speech. Reframing is very similar to the skill you learned earlier about how to modify your irrational, negative thinking. In conversation, this is called "reframing."

If your partner accuses you of lying to her, remember to find truth in her statement. Then you can reframe the idea by disclosing about your own struggle with shame. To do so, you might say something like: "You're right. I was dishonest and I'm sorry for that. I've wanted to tell you for years but I didn't know how. I've recently been figuring out what my fetish is about. I want to share it with you so we can grow closer." See how it's possible to spin something potentially negative into something very positive?

If she says that so much time has been wasted, agree with that. Reframe it this way: "Yes, I agree that we've spent too many years with me being dishonest. I wish it hadn't happened. I'd really like to make up for lost time." Once again, we look at things from another perspective which is fresh and positive.

Many of us react to new situations by saying: "That's too hard for me." I believe it's more helpful to say: "That will be challenging."

Acknowledge Her Efforts

Remember to state your appreciation for her willingness to talk about something difficult. Also remind yourself to say something genuinely affirming to her even if she's oppositional or disagrees with you.

Communicating Your Fetish - A Step-by-Step Guide

You've successfully followed the steps of this program and have come to a place of self-acceptance with your fetish. The process of communication utilizes the same guidelines you followed for yourself. Remember to use your communication skills and to only divulge a little at a time. The slower the better. Don't tell her too much at once. It's not necessary to go into the gory details just yet. There'll be plenty of time for that later. Always give her time to digest and process the information before proceeding to the next step.

Establish achievable goals. Fetish conversation should be taken gradually. You can use the work you've done thus far as your guide. Although the first step for you was education, in this case, with your partner, it will be disclosure. You'll have to tell her that you have a fetish, first and foremost. That will be your initial step. Built into that first disclosure will also be education. You'll have to explain what fetish really means. And, of course, you'll also have to tell her what your fetish actually is. That was your very first question during disclosure. You might want to briefly tell her what your fetish entails.

Initial conversations about fetish should be kept minimal. Further discussion and disclosure will be assessed by her response. Take note of her body language. Does she appear tense and closed off? Relaxed and open? What does she say? Is she interested? Is there any inkling that she thinks this could be fun? Is she receptive? Be very aware of what she says as well as what she doesn't say during these initial conversations.

Step 1 - Education

Once she processes her feelings, she'll be open to hearing the facts about fetish. This is the time to talk about fetish in a general way. You'll teach her the very same things you learned when you first began your journey. Talk about fetish in a very general way. Tell her the definition of fetish. Explain how sexual triggers aren't the same for everyone. Share the websites you found helpful.

But above all, give her as much time and space as she needs to process this. Your patience will ultimately be rewarded. A partner who is willing to do research exhibits some degree of openness. Remember to acknowledge her positive attitude.

Step 2 - Dialoging

In order to encourage real interaction, I want you to know the difference between open-ended versus close-ended questions. Simply put, a close-ended question requires a simple yes or no answer. An open-ended question fosters elaboration upon a topic. Here are examples of each:

Close-Ended Questions:

- At what age did you learn about sex?
- Do you believe in gay marriage?

Open-Ended Questions:

- How did you first learn about sex?
- What was it like for you to find out about sex?
- What are your thoughts and feelings about gay marriage and gay relationships in general?

See how the open-ended questions encourage someone to talk? Close-ended questions quickly end the communication with yes or no responses.

Initial Discussions

Take the lead. I have a feeling you'll be speaking in a way

you've never spoken before. Confidently. About a topic that's probably rarely been discussed. Just initiating these talks gives the message that they are ultra-important not only to you, but to both of you as a couple. She'll get the message!

Start by directing the conversation with an open-ended question. That will guarantee her engagement and participation. In truth, we all like to have the floor. For example you can tell her that you've been thinking about sex in a general way. You're curious to know her opinions and philosophies. What message was she given about sex when she was young? What part of these messages did she adapt as her own? What did she discard? Why does she think sex is an important component of marriage? What does intimacy mean to her?

When it's your turn to speak, model a spirit of being honest and nonjudgmental. The more open you are with her, the more open she'll be with you. Respond to the questions you asked her. Share a little bit about what you were taught concerning sex and marriage.

As your conversation keeps flowing, you can begin to go further and talk about your own unique brand of sexuality, namely fetish. Tell her how you discovered your fetish and how it evolved over the years. Remember to include how it's caused you to feel alone and alienated. Don't leave out the ensuing shame that's led you to be secretive. All of this will help her better understand your fetish and how it's affected you.

Remember that you are still in the initial stage of your talk. I want you to keep the early discussions educational. Don't give her too many details about your fetish right away.

After you do a little disclosing, you can easily segue into a discussion about sex role socialization and societal norms. Think of it like this—in many ways you're building a case and laying a foundation. All of this takes time. Again, don't rush. If she asks a lot of questions about what your fetish entails, she's nervous. Be calm. Be confident. Tell her that you'll get into the specifics later, but for now, you just want to lay the groundwork about fetish in general.

Step 3 - Invite Her In

By now, she's learned that you have a fetish by having

patient, non-threatening discussions about sex and fetish with you. During some of these conversations, you've encouraged her to do research and shared your own knowledge with her. The next step is up to her. Does she want to go further? Hopefully, she will initiate more discussion. If not, you can still act as the catalyst.

Be simple and straightforward. Ask her, "Now that you know about fetish, what do you think?" This is a discussion. Please don't skip over this part. Really talk to her about what she found out. Here's your opportunity to discover what she truly thinks about fetish. Ask her if the educational process has changed her mind in any way. Lead questions might be: "How have your thoughts about fetish changed?" or "In what way has your thinking changed?" and "Do you have any questions about fetish?"

Eventually you will get to the big question, which is: "Do you want to learn more about me and my fetish?" Yes, this is the big question because it could be the "make or break" question for you. Hopefully, she will say yes and you can proceed but if she responds no, you can skip ahead to the next chapter.

Step 4 - Disclosing

Talk about your fetish. Disclose in greater detail how you came to discover your fetish. Try to be as honest and genuine as possible. At this point, she knows about fetish and is clearly curious to learn more about your particular fetish. You're feeling safe enough to tell more.

Now's the time to tell her about your arousal triggers. You can share some of your favorite images and websites at this point. Disclose some of your basic fetish desires. Tell her what it would mean for her to join in with you. Again, you don't have to share everything; just what's necessary. She will need this information so she can make an informed decision about where she'd like to go with this

Step 5 - Checking It Out

Make sure she is hearing you. It may sound strange for me to say this, but remember, you're talking about a charged subject. There's a good chance she's so deep into her own anxiety that she isn't getting a word of what you're saying.

Let's say you've been talking about your craving to be bound and gagged. While you may think you've been speaking eloquently, I bet in her head, she's stuck on the image of you being restrained. She might be worrying about issues like safety, performance and her own sanity. Things that she shouldn't even be thinking about now!

That's why you must draw her back and make sure she's paying attention. The way to do this is to ask her to paraphrase what you've said. You can something like, "So, I just told you that I enjoy being tied up and gagged. Tell me exactly what you heard. This way I'll know you heard me correctly, before we move on."

When I see couples who want to refine their communications skills, I always check their ability to hear their partner correctly. This means one spouse speaks while the other listens. When the speaker if finished, I ask the listener to recap what the other said. The speaker then has the opportunity to make sure they were heard correctly. I encourage you to do this during your fetish discussions.

Again, take this conversation slowly. You don't have to reveal everything in one sitting. Communications should be conveyed in small, bite-sized chunks of information. A little goes a long way. It's entirely possible that she focused on the future and how fetish will impact your lives instead of actually digesting your words. If so, help bring her back to the present. Make sure she understands about the idea of fetish and remind her that the future will be discussed once she can process the nature of fetish in general.

Her feelings also must be addressed. Open-ended questions will allow her to voice any concerns. Find out what's going on inside her head by asking something like: "Now that you've heard about my fetish, how do you feel?" Try to stay on topic and discuss only what you've said thus far. If she wants to know about participation, remind her that you are only talking about the generalities of fetish in the moment. Participation is the next topic.

Be inviting. Always remember to ask her if she's ready to hear more. Sometimes a listener needs a break. A good communicator is always aware of their listener. Encourage her to speak her mind and talk about what she requires from you. Remember to observe her body language, too. Does she appear to be attentive and engaged? If so, then you can move on. Is she fidgety, wringing her hands and looking at the clock? If that's the case, then take a moment to address what you've observed. Ask how she's doing and if necessary, wrap it up for the day. Effective fetish communication should be taken a little at time.

Step 6 - Participation

At this point, she knows you have a fetish. The big question remains: What shall we do about it? Do you want to participate? This is, of course, a mutual decision that you both should weigh in on. It's the admirable, positive way to proceed. She's part of the team.

Don't rush. Don't push. Don't make assumptions. No matter what her reactions to your disclosures have been, she needs time to process them and think things over.

Even if you guess that she's not interested, you still have to ask the question. This is the only way to get a definitive answer. It also invites more participation, respect and discussion. Don't be discouraged if she initially says that she doesn't want to participate. This response might mean she's still unsure. A good communicator always probes, checks out comments and is open to deeper discussion.

Step 7 - Sharing the Details of Your Personal Identification

Here's the best-case scenario. You've bared your "fetish soul" and her answer is affirmative! Yes, she wants to join with you and participate. She doesn't know what this entails, but she's ready to learn more. Lucky you!

Does that mean you should immediately get out your clothing, props or sex toys and head directly for the bedroom? Hell, no. Remember, she's a complete newcomer when it comes to your fetish and fetish fulfillment. Share with her only the very basics of your Identification Process at this point.

Step 8 - What to Do First

Great! She wants to participate with you—now what? For starters, do something easy and basic. For example, if you have a foot fetish, you can begin by taking off her shoes and kissing her bare feet. If you have a fetish for panties, have her put on her favorite pair and model them for you. Remember to proceed with caution. You don't want to scare her off but to gradually, gently introduce her to your fetish.

If your fetish calls for some kind of physical interaction, start by doing something to her very, very, very lightly. If it's bondage, take a pair of her hose and loosely tie her hands above her head. Make sure you do this in an extremely erotic manner. Employ sensuality whether it's your real scene or not. It's a perfect, gentle, caring way to introduce her to your fetish. Right now, your main goal is to create positive feelings attached to your fetish.

If you're into spanking, even if you prefer to be spanked, it's a good idea to spank her first. Do it softly and voluptuously, lighter than light. Remember that spanking fetishist I mentioned in Chapter 12? The one who put on music, eased his wife over his lap and tapped her bottom to the beat? Notice that I said tap! He was careful not to strike her anywhere near as harshly as he likes. Again, these initial encounters are meant to create positive associations with the fetish, so it's importantly to tread lightly.

Step 9 - Going Deeper

As you and your partner get comfortable, you can slowly but surely introduce her to the more intricate details of your fetish. Each time something new is introduced, remember to check in with her first. You can do this by asking things like: "How do you feel hearing about this?" or "Is this something you think you'd be comfortable to try with me?"

Any time you and she interact or play, you must also communicate. It doesn't have to be at the moment you're done but at some point before you move forward in your fetish play. Hopefully, you're both satisfied and fall into a deep, relaxing slumber afterwards. However, at some point, you do want to check in. To do so, ask her: "How was the fetish play for you?," Did you have fun?" and "Is there anything you'd like to talk about?"

Likewise, she has to communicate with you as well. Especially if she's the top and is dominating you. She'll need your feedback about how she's orchestrating the scene.

But it's important that you two actually do things to each other, whatever they are. For example, if it's bondage you're into, find a pair of stockings and tie up her legs or vice versa. If you like D/s, make love with her on top. Invite her to give you instructions on how to please her orally. If your fetish is more detailed, go online and purchase some kind of implement or sex toy together.

The more you play, the better it will be and the more comfortable you will both be about exploring the parameters of your fetish together.

Step 10 - The Talking Alternative

Some of your identified fetish needs might be way too complicated or uncomfortable for her to engage in with you. But don't despair. And don't keep secrets. Many fetishists love hearing about their fetish while masturbating. You can offer her verbiage, acts and scenarios from your inner fantasy life. Though they might be outrageous, sharing them with her brings her into your world.

If she's willing to participate in fantasy talk with you, she now becomes an integral part of your fetish world. She becomes a facilitator. As a result, you will gain a greater sense of intimacy. She knows your secrets and what makes you tick, and is happy to be part of the "ticking."

Stranger than Fiction

You just never know what will happen when your wife learns about your fetish. I just read an article in The Washington Post about a woman who decided to stay with her husband David when he became Deborah after a sex-change operation. If you wish to read it yourself, search the Washington Post. The article ran on August 19, 2014.

Leslie Hilburn Fabian even wrote a book about the experience, My Husband's a Woman Now: A Shared Journey of Transition and Love. Leslie met her husband in 1991 when he was dressed as a woman at a party. Though David sometimes cross-dressed, he lived as a man...and was a successful New England surgeon, in fact. After 20 years of marriage, David realized that he wanted more, and his wife loved him so much that she decided to stay by his side and stay married.

So, you never know until you share your story with your spouse. There are stranger stories out there than yours! Of course, the tale of David/Deborah and Leslie is extreme but it is true. It's living, breathing testimony of what can happen if you're honest with your spouse about your fetish desires.

In Summary

Effective communication is a skill that can be developed and learned. All couples must understand how to communicate in order to maintain a relationship.

Communication is vital if you're choosing to introduce fetish into your relationship. There's never any guarantee that your partner will be open to participation. However, you stand a much better chance of gaining her acceptance if you utilize the basic communication skills I've outlined for you here.

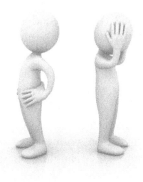

Chapter 18 - What If She Still Says No?

Up until now, you've been sailing along nicely. You've come to a place of understanding, and are not only exploring but are accepting yourself and your fetish. You thought long and hard about the pros and cons of disclosure. You considered the possibility that she won't be able to comprehend your fetish, but in the end, you decided to give it a shot. Pat yourself on the back because this demonstrates a large amount of positivity about your character. You are direct, honest and want to be open. This holds true even if you've withheld telling her for years.

Now that you've come to a place of confidence, you feel it's best to be forthright. Your wishes are altruistic and unselfish. You want to be more candid with your mate. You'd like to be closer and more intimate with the one you love. That's very commendable.

You did your best to communicate your longings with her. You followed the guidelines laid out in this book and practiced patience. However, despite your best your efforts, your woman is still negative about your fetish. You may be feeling sad, rejected or even angry. You're probably telling yourself that you'll never get your needs met, that you're unlovable or it's not fair that you were "cursed" with a fetish.

Remember, your emotions are linked with your thoughts, so it's time to think differently. You're the same great guy you've always been, aren't you? You're a good, caring partner. You chose to share your fetish with your partner with the hopes of coming clean and growing closer. Her reaction is not reflective of you, your character or the fact that you have a fetish. She's rejecting your fetish because of her own belief system about sex and what intimacy should or shouldn't be about. Her feelings aren't necessarily what's right; they're just what are.

Even after listening to you, your partner still didn't hear you. Why? Because she's caught up in what she thinks to be true about sexuality. She's a product of society. Fetish is something foreign to her. As a result, she had a spontaneous, negative reaction. In her mind, the idea of fetish and fantasy is inherently wrong, perverse and unacceptable. She's a black-and-white thinker, i.e. she believes that sex has to be one way or another. It's a penis penetrating a vagina, and that's it. She wants nothing to do with your fetish and she wants it out of her life. Period. The end.

But please don't feel dejected. You don't have to give up—unless you choose to do so. If you still want to have her join in your fetish with you, try to get a handle on your fetish from her point of view. Don't despair; get prepared.

Right now, I'm going to give you the top reasons why women are opposed to fetish, D/s and other sexual behaviors that are out of the norm. With better understanding, you'll gain greater empathy. These insights will also help you deepen future discussions. It's not over yet. In many ways, it's just beginning.

Here's what your woman may be thinking:

Common Reasons for Saying No

Your fetish is not manly.

That's a very true statement, especially if your fetish calls for you to take on the submissive role. She's absolutely correct in a very traditional, antiquated way of thinking. Sex-role socialization is a powerful concept that most women buy into, especially when it comes to bedroom activities. She's been brought up to think about men as masculine creatures. The image is primal, almost caveman-like. The traditional male is supposed to be strong, decisive and provide for their families. In the bedroom, their role is to take the lead. Even if she intellectually knows differently, sexually she's programmed to believe otherwise; it's taken years and years of conditioning.

But the above mentioned belief is a fallacy and an incorrect, stereotypical way of thinking. Fortunately for you, we are living in a time when women are taking on sexy, superhero roles. Think of Catwoman, Wonder Woman, Supergirl and a host of others. Think of the actresses who play bad asses—Lucy Lui, Angelina Jolie or Mia Kirshner. These women are no-nonsense, independent and accomplished. In movie scripts, they take the lead. Slowly but surely, the mindset about what's sexy and feminine is changing. In the future, I think the idea of female dominance won't even be an issue. Ultimately, we want men and women to be in touch with both sides of their personalities. This means you both have the opportunity to exercise your dominant and submissive sides in the bedroom.

Your fetish is chauvinistic.

Sometimes it seems like you just can't win! If you lean more toward being dominant, she will probably object to that as well. She'll say your ideas are antiquated and old-fashioned. She'll remind you that she's equal to you both in and out of the boudoir.

Basically, the reason for this is she's frightened and doesn't want to lose control. She's also afraid that you might get carried away and hurt her. This is actually something you can easily work on if she allows her mindset to change.

Role-playing might be a fun way to go. It will give you the opportunity to release yourselves from "politically correct" ideas and get into character. Traditional D/s people will opt for Master/slave roles. But you can also adapt roles of leader and subordinate such as teacher/student, boss/secretary or policeman/thief.

Your fetish objectifies me.

This is the Number One fetish deal-breaker. It's also the biggest argument made women make against fetish. The very word "objectify" gives her refusal validity. But that's not necessarily what's going on. It's really about her own discomfort with sexual variation, not so much about your fetish.

Here's an example of the objectification argument in action:

Mike met Sue on an Internet dating site. He was initially attracted to her because she wore leather in her profile picture. They met, hit it off and the relationship soon grew serious. One day, Mike disclosed to Sue why he liked her picture. He took a deep breath and admitted that he had a boot fetish. Then he presented her with a pair of gorgeous thigh-high boots. Sue wore them and they proceeded to have passionate sex.

Fast-forward two years. Sue doesn't want to wear the boots any longer. Instead, she opts for sweat pants. Why? Because she feels wearing boots objectifies her, that Mike's more interested in the boots than he is in her. Sue wants Mike to be attracted to her and not the boots. To dispel this one-sided mode of thinking, Mike has to convince Sue that she's the one who turns him on; boots are just the icing on the cake.

You care more for your fetish than you do for me.

This is another common argument women have against fetish. Women like to be the center of attention. (And who doesn't?) They want you to be attracted to them and only them. They reason that if you have a fetish, you're more into your object, act or scenario than you are to them. They want you to be excited only by their presence. They feel that fetish is their competition. And they don't like having to compete for your affection, whether it be competing with another person or a rubber beach ball.

Your fetish lowers the value of sex.

Our culture tells us that sex is about intimacy, and intimacy comes in but one form: conventional, traditional foreplay followed by standard (usually missionary-style) intercourse. Fetish veers off this trusty, tried-and-true path. The Bible wouldn't approve and neither does your partner. She will conveniently pull out this line of reasoning and use it as an excuse not to engage with you and your fetish. But the truth is that she probably doesn't like anything different or threatening. Your fetish is scary and off-putting for her.

Your fetish causes you to be distant.

Sexual gurus speak volumes about being "present" during sex. Your wife might be one who has embraced this concept. If so, you will be faced with her argument that fetish is distancing. She will argue that you're more involved with the fetish than you are with her. She will have the voice of spiritual and religious teachings to back her ideals. While you can find the truth in her misgivings about fetish, there are also deeper truths that you know to be more realistic. The truths you've learned in this book, for example.

Your partner wants sex to be a totally present lovemaking experience. She wants you to look into her eyes and focus only on her and how beautiful she is to you. From your point of view, she would be even more beautiful in leather, latex or hose but this is contrary to her belief about how sex "should be." It should be all about her and not costuming, an act or verbiage. Your fetish conflicts with her ideal. She will say that it takes away from your intimacy.

Actually, sharing a lifelong secret that previously caused you shame and embarrassment is the ultimate form of closeness. And you'll be looking at her with an unimaginable intimacy and devotion while enacting your fetish if only she'd give it a chance. But instead, she fears your fetish makes you distant.

Here's another vignette to illustrate this particular mode of thought:

Jason enjoys BDSM interplay and wanted to include his wife. He didn't want this type of play every time they had sex but he thought it would be awesome if Lily would participate every now and again. But instead of having an open mind about it, she said "no" immediately as almost a knee-jerk reaction. Her excuse? Her spirituality.

Lily was incredibly judgmental about the whole concept of D/s exchanges. She felt that this kind of interplay wasn't sexy and couldn't understand the notion of pain as being pleasurable. As a result, Lily shut out her husband because his fantasy didn't conform with her rigid concept of intimacy. Even worse, she quizzed him about his thoughts every time they were in the middle of having "vanilla" sex. Lily accused his mind of of being elsewhere while they were having relations.

And do you know what happened? Eventually, Jason did indeed go elsewhere. Right into the stockades of a professional Dominatrix who was happy to fulfill his needs—for a fee. If Lily had explored and educated herself about BDSM, she would have discovered that this kind of interplay is as intense as it is mind-expanding. It's as spiritual as it is sensual. BDSM can be astounding and powerful. It can make tantric sex look like an outdated 1950s marital primer.

Sex is about variety and having different experiences. Real-time presence is great but so is fantasy and role-play. True, sex may be about lots of foreplay, oral sex and presence, but these are in no way mandatory. You can be "present" within the context of fetish play as well.

Rigid spouses are only looking at one side of the issue. They present themselves as being sexually open when in fact, they are old-fashioned and narrow-minded. Hours of passionate lovemaking may be all well and good, but if you're a fetishist, they'll never be as exciting as the fetish itself. These are solid facts that your woman will have to learn if she wants to have a real, whole, honest relationship with you.

Your fetish is selfish.

Sometimes, women argue that fetish is selfish. They say that it's all about you: "Why should I have to do the things he wants?" or "Why should I do things to him when he should be doing things to me?"

Why indeed?! That's a very good point. But she should also be asking herself the same question. It's pretty selfish not to want to participate in something that would make you happy. In the past, you probably bought into this notion. You used to think that fetish was self-indulgent, but not anymore. You now understand that you're not asking for something "extra." You're talking about a desire that's genuine and real, something powerful that will never go away. You have a profound longing to indulge your fetish in a safe, sane way. I wouldn't define that as "extra;" I'd call it vital.

At its very foundation, marriage is about compromise. Many of the activities you do together are things that you'd never do if you were single but you do them for her. You go to the mall, run errands and go out with her friends because that makes her happy. Maybe you'd rather stay home and watch the game but you do these little things to show her that you care.

Likewise, sexual satisfaction is about compromise. No one gets pleasure at the exact same moment. One partner might prefer the woman-on-top position while the other likes doggie-style best of all. Think about oral sex. The giver is never feeling as much pleasure as the receiver, yet we perform oral sex to make our partners happy. Ultimately, in a good, strong marriage, you want to be pleasing to each other. It's a two-way street.

Your fetish is perverse.

By labeling your fetish as perverse, your partner simply detaches. She writes off your fetish based on a word that really describes unconventionality. In her book, anything that deviates from the norm is labeled as wrong. And she reasons, "If it's wrong, then I don't have to engage." This is a foolproof reasoning in that it allows her to excuse herself from your fetish.

Real-Life Examples

Here are a couple of real-life examples of what I'm referring to:

Brent has a strong panty fetish. He'd often give his wife, Carla, beautiful panties for Christmas and Valentine's Day. When she wore them, he'd get very excited and Brent would be more amorous than usual. He would especially love performing oral sex on Carla while she wore the panties he gave her.

One day, Brent mustered the courage to admit that he had a passion for panties. Carla overreacted by never wearing any of the panties he gave her as gifts again. Then, when Carla found out that Brent sometimes liked to wear panties himself, she made sure to trash every Victoria's Secret catalog as soon as it arrived. She felt her husband was perverted and sick.

Similarly, Doug likes to masturbate while holding a pair of silky stockings. His wife, Amy, caught him and said she'd divorce him if she ever saw that type of behavior again. This is another strong reaction by a wife who tells herself that anything sexual she perceives as out of the norm must be rejected.

Unfortunately, Carla and Amy are dismissing the facts about fetish. Their refusal to open their minds to the concept of fetish just may cause them to harm their marriage. They hide behind a word instead of opening themselves up to new possibilities.

What does "perverted" mean anyway? According to the Merriam-Webster Dictionary, the word "perverted" means "having or showing sexual desires that are considered not normal or acceptable." Notice that the definition said "considered." Who makes up these rules anyway? Who creates the norm? We know the answer. Society, religion our parents. There's no real credibility from any of these areas. They're only beliefs by people who aren't true thinkers. They're "followers" who don't know how to form their own ideas or opinions.

Another important point is that Carla and Amy fail to let themselves understand the truth. And that truth is that their husbands want to see *them* wearing the clothing. They don't want to see someone else wearing it. They could be the object of their husband's lust and they're treating it carelessly.

The same goes for you and your lady. You would prefer to participate in your fetish with your partner. You would also give anything to have her acceptance and she just doesn't get how important this is to you—or your relationship in general.

Wives like Carla and Amy choose to stick to their ideas rather than learn the facts about fetish. They both would rather be "right" than loved. They have access to the knowledge that would make them an incredible lover in their husband's eyes. They own the key to his heart and were entrusted with privileged information. They could have their hot little hands on the insurance policy that would guarantee total fidelity. Instead, they choose to disregard the information and reject instead of accept. Sue, Carla, Amy and Lily, and many other uninformed wives have chosen being "right" over being loved.

What Do You Do Now?

It's extremely difficult to change someone's mode of thought. Think about how difficult it was for you to change the way you felt about your fetish. You must be patient with her initial reactions. Now that you're feeling unapologetic about your fetish, this could very well change important dynamics in your relationship.

Let's take a moment to look at where we are at this juncture. Your partner has had an initial, negative gut reaction to your communication about your fetish. She strongly identifies with one or more of the objections I've just outlined previously. The question is: Would she rather be right? Or would she rather be close to you? Would she like true intimacy in her marriage or would she prefer that you compartmentalize it? Compartmentalization is an option but ultimately, it draws couples apart rather than bring them closer together.

Now's a good time to remind yourself that you have a fetish that is strong, powerful and doesn't go away. It probably was part of your life long before your partner was. Your fetish needs must be fed. Much like cooking at home or going out to a restaurant, your woman can choose to do the feeding herself or you can do it on your own. Or pay someone else to make your fetish "meals."

I often work with wives of fetishists and use the example below which is usually very helpful. I call it "The Vibrator Argument." Feel free to share it with her or to come up with something similar on your own. I call it:

The Vibrator Argument

Many women have trouble achieving orgasm, especially from regular intercourse. Since the beginning of time, women struggled with the fact that men didn't really understand female anatomy. Within the past 50 years or so, the feminist movement has brought to light the fact that women have a clitoris, and that it's been ignored by men for centuries. Believe it or not, before then, most people (men and women) were not that aware of this part of the vagina, this little piece of skin above the opening which holds the nerves that cause excitement. Think of the clitoris as the female penis. Clitoral stimulation is necessary in order for a female to have an orgasm. Men were sorry to hear this. They thought it was their penis going in and out of the vagina that did the trick. But women were elated because they now knew what it took to get them over the edge.

Anatomically, it's often impossible for women to achieve orgasm solely through intercourse alone. Therefore, manual or oral stimulation is required. Many men were too tired—or in too much of a hurry—to do this every time. Is it much of a surprise that the vibrator was born? The vibrator is referred to by many as a girl's best friend. Your partner can probably relate.

Maybe your wife is one of these women who loves her vibrator and relies on this handy, little device to achieve orgasm. Ask her how she would feel if you suddenly decided that vibrators were sick or wrong—it should be your penis and your penis alone that makes her orgasm. Imagine if you took away her vibrator. She'd probably feel very frustrated and resentful as well as incredibly tense.

Now, tell her to imagine that she had to hide her vibrator and use it only on the sly, when you weren't around. What if you found it one day and got angry. Or if you humiliated her because you walked in on her pleasuring herself with a vibrator? How would she feel? Especially if you told all of her friends. That awful, frustrated, angry feeling is exactly what you feel when she doesn't allow you to engage in your fetish. And it's not her participation you're asking for; it's her acceptance.

Fetish Can Be About Her

Sue, Carla, Lily and Amy all felt justified in withholding their partners' objects of desire. They failed to understand the very essence of their men's disclosure. In each case, their husbands wanted to integrate them into their fetish. Participation would allow them to get closer to their respective mates. Instead, they drove their partners away.

Similarly, many professionals in the psychological community will preach intimacy and see fetish play as the opposite. What they don't understand is that the fetish is a part of you that won't disappear. It's absolutely detrimental to you that they provide ammunition with words like "objectification" and provide unhelpful diagnoses such as "paraphilia." Your partners use these words as a way to distance themselves from your fetish, to excuse themselves from it. The terms provide a justification for their fears. It's always easier to reject the unknown than to embrace it.

Sexual relations are difficult to maintain in any long-term relationship. The fact that you have a fetish actually makes erotic encounters pretty easy—after all, you have something dependable that rings your bell, no matter what. Your wife has to really understand this point. She must embrace it. It's key that she understand she has access to a magical button which she can push at any time that will always get you aroused. It's no longer a mystery. She knows what to say to you. She knows what to do to you. You've told her and you can disclose more, if only she were willing. All she has to do is change her thinking a little bit more and her reward will be a happy, content husband who will not stray. What you're asking isn't impossible.

Aim Toward Acceptance

If she says no, you have to decide how to proceed. At this point, you feel accepting of your fetish but an essential piece of that puzzle isn't intact. How will you live with someone who is rejecting a key component of your sexuality?

Now that you're more aware of her objections, it's time to address them. You must probe deeper and find out what her real fears are. Are you really objectifying her? Putting your fetish first? Is there is any truth in her objections? If so, acknowledge them. Maybe you're too overzealous about having to incorporate fetish activity every single time you have sex. If so, why not pull back a bit and see how this goes?

Fighting Back

First, acknowledge that your partner has some good points about fetish. It's true that your fetish might go against traditional gender expectations, be a little off-putting and be difficult for her to associate with feelings of sexual arousal. She can argue those points for days—and they're valid points to make.

But in the end, recognize that your fetish is your sexual trigger. She can choose to be accepting or she can choose to be rejecting. I've met and counseled a large number of men with wives who gave their fetish a thumbs-down. A few even gave ultimatums like "Drop the fetish or drop me!" These men were good men and didn't want to break up the family unit so they agreed with their wives' decree. But the results weren't usually what the ladies had in mind.

For Example...

Take Jeff, for instance. Jeff had a fetish for angora sweaters. He'd buy them on eBay and accrued a quite a huge collection. He'd wear them at home and would masturbate while holding the garment in his hand. His wife Maria always thought his fetish was some kind of strange quirk. After Jeff started doing some work on self-acceptance, he decided to come clean about the fetish and told his all about it. He actually followed the steps I provided and did an impressive job communicating his fetish with her. Still, Maria said the fetish was a no-go. Not only did she refuse to wear a sweater as Jeff requested but she angrily discarded his whole collection one day while Jeff was at work.

Understandably, Jeff was devastated by his wife's reaction but he also felt his wife was more important to him than angora sweaters. This was a noble gesture that didn't work. Why? Because as time went on Jeff felt angry and resentful. He started to spend less time at home and more time socializing with friends. Eventually, he struck up a friendship with a woman who thought the idea of wearing angora sweaters was fun and kinky. You can guess what happened from there.

Let me tell you a bit about Tony. He had a fetish for smothering. All it required was that his wife sit on his face and suffocate him for a second or two with her bottom. He also liked the idea of being farted upon while tonguing her anus. There were elements of D/s, control and humiliation contained in his fetish. Sounds simple enough, right?

But Poor Tony never got past the smothering part. His wife Tanya rejected and humiliated him. She even told her friends about his very personal fetish. Tony felt mortified and ashamed. But he also had already gained self-compassion. He understood that his fetish was but one small part of his being. Tony also decided to drop the idea of fetish with his wife and get his needs met elsewhere. He enjoyed time alone on the computer exploring his fetish and went to the occasional session with a professional sex worker. Tony never talked about his fetish with Tanya again. So far, the marriage has lasted but there's underlying tension within this couple's relationship. I don't think the overall prognosis is good.

Take a look at Kenneth. He also has a fetish for smothering and squashing. He loves the idea of a big-bootied woman sitting on his face—and sitting on it hard. As a result, he's always dated large-sized women. When Kenneth met Polly, he knew she was the one. Polly was warm, funny, caring and had a very large bottom. Kenneth was thrilled but he was also reluctant to share his fetish with Polly. He worried that she'd think he chose to be with her just for her big behind. Kenneth knew his relationship with Polly was strong besides his fascination with her glorious bottom. They were kind and thoughtful with each other, had many shared interests and were deeply in love. Of course, Polly was aware of Kenneth's preference for big booty but she was comfortable with herself and with her "ass"ets. She liked who she was and that included her voluptuous derriere.

When Kenneth finally shared his overall fetish for smothering and squashing, Polly was intrigued. She wanted to know more. She was inquisitive and open to learning how to please Kenneth. One day, he had her climb on top of him. Polly knew he was in heaven by his bodily reaction. She felt thrilled to be able to provide so much pleasure to her man. This, in turn, gave her pleasure.

Kenneth and Polly have been married for almost a decade. Smothering is still a part of their bedroom activities in between raising a family, building successful careers and remaining blissfully in love. Polly knows Kenneth's fetish is unusual, and her response is, "So what! Everyone has their stuff. I'm just glad that my big booty got me the husband I always wanted."

Polly is a woman who's open to new experiences. She didn't have expectations about what Kenneth "should be" in terms of sex. She merely accepted him for who he was and actually enjoyed the fact that she could provide pleasure with a part of her body that many would consider to be too fat or too big. As a result, she has a happy life and a happy husband. She doesn't have expectations about the people in her life, but instead, takes them as they are with a loving attitude of acceptance.

Maria and Tanya paid the price for intolerance. They both thought they were "right." They both got validation from friends, therapists and colleagues who advised them not to put up with their partners' perverse behaviors. They thought they were teaching their men a lesson by not engaging in fetish play. But who wins in the end? Both women are left with unhappy mates who physically or emotionally leave. Is it worth it for them to "be right?" Wouldn't it be better if they had taken the time to learn more about their husbands' fetish and at least try to embrace them?

I know that at this point, you might be feeling like Jeff or Tony. You might be thinking, 'It's not worth it. She'll never change.' You might stick around because of your commitment to your wife and your family. But what about your commitment to yourself? You night even try to forget your fetish and even your sexuality in an attempt to make things right. But you'll do so resentfully. Even worse, you'll keep hoping your life could be more like Kenneth's. And you'll feel regretful that you didn't pick a Polly.

Beware of remorse or of "going back." Remember all the reasons you're with your partner. Think back to the day you met her and when you fell in love. She's still the same special lady. It might be worth it to keep trying to get her to understand and accept your fetish. It might be worth it to gift her a copy of my book *Sex, Fetish and Him*, to educate her more about fetish, to show her she isn't alone and that the phenomenon isn't uncommon. I discuss the book more deeply at the end of this chapter.

Only you will know whether or not you should pursue it. If you do, remember the essential components that will lead her toward joining with you in your fetish:

Refresher Course: Key Communication Components

Understanding

Just like you, she must educate herself on the nature of sexual fetish. She has to understand that a high percentage of the population enjoys some kind of sexual activity that is considered "out of the norm." If so many people enjoy this, it stands to reason that it's more normal than abnormal. With understanding comes desensitization. The more she understands, the less freaky your fetish will appear to her. It will be normalized for her.

Acceptance

She has to change her thinking. Instead of seeing you as being abnormal, she has to think of you as having an unusual need. Instead of thinking that this fetish is drawing you apart, she has to understand that this fetish can draw you together in a big way. You must open up and let her see how difficult it's been for you to have this fetish. Share the struggles you've had and the journey you've taken toward self-acceptance. Share that you are proud of your own accomplishments. Make sure she understands that you will never return to a place of secrecy and shame. You've gotten to your destination and you want her to get to the same place. Only then, will you really join together and have the type of intimate marriage that you both deserve. Let her know that you would like—and prefer—her support but you will never acquiesce to feeling bad about your fetish.

Acceptance will sustain your health, mental and otherwise. When you feel anxious about your fetish, you will act out in a compulsive, disordered fashion—like masturbating incessantly. But instead, you have made a commitment toward health. Her support would be helpful but if she's not on board you will do what it takes to stay healthy. Meaning, you will seek fulfillment with a professional or on the Internet, whatever it takes.

Retrain Her Brain

Talk to her about changing her way of thinking about your fetish. This will also make her feel better about herself. She will feel like she chose wisely in you. She will understand that fetish is only one small component of who you are as a human being. Accepting this small but different piece of you will help her know that she truly loves you for who you are; not who she hoped you would be.

Love is unconditional and your self-esteem is now high enough that you require love in the true sense of the word—fully, deeply, totally. In turn, you will love her in that very same unconditional way. No one is perfect and I'm sure she knows that she has her own quirks as well, and that you love and accept her in spite of them.

Is Fetish Cause for Divorce?

This is a very weighty, life-changing question. The response is extremely personal and individualized—and entirely up to you. Can you live with your wife not accepting your fetish? Can you remain close to her without harboring resentment? Can you accept a woman who doesn't accept you fully? Do you want to?

The marriages that broke up might have been triggered by fetish but there is always something more. Fetish was merely the tip of the iceberg. A spouse who's controlling, selfish and argumentative about fetish will be that way in other areas of the relationship as well. (I know a wife who says, "I'm never wrong," and wholeheartedly believes it! Take it from me, no one is never wrong.) Sometimes these behaviors will be highlighted during fetish discussions. You will notice them because these heart-to-hearts are so important to you. In reality, these negative behaviors have always been present in your spouse but fetish brings them to the surface and makes them even more evident.

Many of you have families you want to keep intact. And most of you have partners that you love very much. It's just "this fetish thing" which has caused a wedge between you. This is why I encourage you to modify your communications style and keep going. Try to voice your desires and the importance of your fetish without hounding her, yet getting her to understand it, and hopefully, to accept it.

Try and Try Again

If she says no, it's important not to give up. Ask yourself how you communicated about fetish the last time? Did you take your time? Did you give her enough time to think and process? Did you introduce only a little bit of information at a time? One discussion about fetish is never enough. This is a process. It's something you've been dealing with all your life. She needs time to grasp your revelation. Don't lose heart.

Sex, Fetish and Him

Unfortunately, I've met many women like Maria and Tanya. So many, in fact, that they inspired me to write my book, Sex, Fetish and Him. Women like Tanya and Maria have many incorrect beliefs about fetish. They believe that fetish is a disease. They think any kind of sexuality that can't be neatly cubby-holed is wrong or perverse. They go on to mislabel their husbands' fetish as addictive behavior. They think that treatment will "cure" them of their affliction.

Instead of educating themselves, these women respond to their husbands' attempts to explain their fetish with a litany of unkind messages. They label their husbands as sick, perverted and weird. They want to have nothing to do with the fetish. They are rejecting and turn their backs on their men. Then, these very same women are surprised when their husbands withdraw, resent them or seek pleasure elsewhere.

The misguided reactions by otherwise caring wives are truly toxic. Yes, a sexual fetish is different. But it doesn't make you sick or wrong. It means that you have something quirky that happens to produce arousal. The fetish doesn't change who you are. You are still the wonderful guy they married and chose to spend the rest of their lives with. Your women are simply uneducated. Like you, they have to understand and then change their way of thinking. Until they do so, they will have a knee-jerk reaction to your fetish. Their "Gospel truths" about sex turn out to be outright lies and contrary to what you require as a fetishist.

At the very least, *Sex, Fetish and Him* will be an educational tool to school your wife even more deeply about fetish, and hopefully, set her out on the road to acceptance.

In Summary

Your marriage is worth fighting for. I believe every marriage is. So is your self-esteem. There has to be a win/win solution and this is reached through compromise. If she says no, don't get discouraged. Give her time to process what you've told her and then ease your way into the discussion again. And again. Whatever it takes.

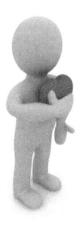

Chapter 19 - Healthy Incorporation

We're nearing the end of our journey. I'll bet that at some points, you didn't think you'd make it this far. But you did and I'm very proud of your perseverance and determination.

At this juncture, you know the definition of fetish. You have an understanding of what your own fetish entails. Most importantly, you've come to a place of realization about your fetish. You've been thoughtful about what it would take to get your fetish wishes met. Now it's time to consider your options and figure out how to incorporate fetish into your life in a healthy way.

Healthy fetish incorporation means acknowledging the fact that you have a fetish. As such, you recognize that you have specific needs. Although these needs must be met, they do not have to take precedence over your other basic human needs. Instead, they must be recognized and incorporated into your life in a balanced way. Fetish desires are not given greater or lesser importance than any of your other desires. You now know that you are a dynamic human being and that you are not defined by your fetish.

Part of self-acceptance means that fetish no longer has to be your "dirty little secret." Nor do you have to exert mountains of energy trying to repress an important component of your sexuality. Given the idea that your fetish is strong, powerful and will never go away, let's consider your options:

1. You can keep your fetish as a solitary activity.

Your fetish is yours. You have worked through your negative feelings and can finally admit that you enjoy your fetish. It gives you pleasure. It's a catalyst for your sexual release. And best of all, now that you've shed your shame and embarrassment, you can fully enjoy your fantasies anxiety free.

You've done your due diligence and know exactly what it would take to enact your fantasy with another human being. However, you've come to the conclusion that your fetish is too intricate and complicated to share with another person. You might have also tried to communicate your needs to your significant other only to be met with opposition.

As a result of all of the above, you've decided that you do not want to go outside of your marriage and feel that you can get your fetish wishes met on your own. Whatever your reasoning, you have arrived at a place where you're choosing to keep your fetish activity solitary. And most importantly, you're all right with this decision.

Making up your mind to keep your fetish as an alone activity, doesn't mean that you push your feelings aside or under the rug. It simply means that you are choosing to fantasize by yourself. Notice the word "choosing." That word is important. This is your choice.

Solitary fetish activity can include masturbation by yourself while you think of your fetish. It can also include masturbating online while watching images or video clips dedicated to your specific fetish.

If there is a material, object or piece of clothing that you find arousing, you can include these articles in your solo fetish exploration without shame or guilt. This means that as a panty fetishist, you'll allow yourself the pleasure of wearing panties. Or as a mohair sweater fetishist, you'll collect—and wear—your favorite sweaters. If you like to masturbate while holding lingerie, you will do so. You will allow yourself time to engage in your fetish without feeling bad about yourself.

This being said, you will also take heed of others. You will not engage in behaviors that might be inappropriate or risky. Meaning, that if you wear panties outside of the house, you'll wear them under your clothes. You will be cognizant of when to wear them and never put them on if there's any risk of someone seeing you (like wearing them to the gym, for instance). You will be respectful of other people and never allow strangers to question your intentions or make others feel uncomfortable. This is about being appropriate and considerate of others, in addition to recognizing your own wants.

If your wife is opposed to your activities, you will be as discrete as possible when enacting your fetish in private. Masturbation will take place at times when you would be alone—not when she's home and simply in another room. Again, you will be respectful of her feelings and not be at your computer viewing fetish images when you could be in bed with her. This is also to protect yourself from her disdain as well as being responsible in your marriage.

At the same time, you will not allow your wife or partner to dictate what is right or wrong for you. If she doesn't understand your fetish, that's her personal issue, not yours. Although she doesn't have to participate, she simply cannot take away your need for fetish fulfillment. She has no right to control what you think about no more than you have a right to control her thoughts.

Remember that acknowledging your fetish provides you with the same kind of pleasure as getting lost in a book, going for a long run or going for a relaxing drive down a peaceful country road. It's a way to escape and distract yourself from the grind of everyday life. Just do it within reason. The general rule of thumb about fetish and masturbation is that it's absolutely healthy as long it doesn't interfere with your family, friends or spouse. In other words, you're not leaving the cocktail party to go home and play with yourself.

If you engage in fetish masturbation in a way that's equivalent to watching a favorite TV show, participating in sports or a hobby, then you're within reason and it's your right to do this. Your fetish should be a time-limited activity, not an obsession. If you find yourself losing track of the hours, take note. You might find it useful to set the timer on your phone so you remember to disengage at an appropriate point.

But by all means, allow yourself to enjoy your solitary fetish time. It's your right. It's your need. Enjoy it and luxuriate in it!

2. You can compartmentalize.

Compartmentalization means that you would like to participate in fetish play with a consenting adult who is separate and apart from your day-to-day life. You've chosen this option based upon your fetish identification and the communication you did (or didn't have) with your significant other. You've decided that your fetish will best be met outside of your primary relationship.

Some of you may even be single and you've decided that you don't want to share your fetish within the context of a long-term, primary relationship. As long as you have consciously made this decision with a mindset of self-acceptance, that's fine. The choice is always yours. It's your life and you must live it the way that's best for you.

Often people from cultures outside the U.S. choose this option. So do very religious people. No matter how much they try, they know that fetish will conflict with the mentality of their culture. They know it would be impossible to explain their fetish to a future partner, so in the end, they know that compartmentalization works best. It's easiest for everyone in their lives, but especially, for themselves. They've discovered wonderful options to indulge in their fetish, which include:

Websites and Social Media

If you are single and have chosen to compartmentalize, you have a number of possibilities open to you. Of course, you still have your favorite websites. You also have online fetish communities. Many fetishists enjoy chat rooms, private chats, webcams and telephone conversations. You can talk about the fetish or even have mutual fetish/fantasy sex talk. You enjoy the advantage of chatting within the privacy of your own home. This is a very easy, safe, inexpensive way to interact with someone else and never leave your house. Besides not being dangerous, it's fun and cost-effective.

Some of you will choose to extend electronic chats to in-person meetings. The purpose of getting together would only be for fetish play. My advice is to engage in face-to-face fetish play, if you've talked to that person for an extended time and feel confident that they are a compatible match.

Some of you will choose to meet for a cup of coffee first and schedule play time for another date. Others will want to dive right in. Whatever your choice, please use common sense. The Internet is an absolutely fantastic tool for bringing fetishists together, however, people are not always what they appear to be while chatting online or even speaking on the telephone. It's always best to meet somewhere public at first to talk more about your fetish. Be sure to establish safety guidelines. Let someone you trust know who you're meeting and where. Check in with this friend during the meeting with your potential fetish playmate and let that friend know you're safe.

I realize I'm talking to men right now, but many guys get fooled, too. Remember the mini-scandals when actor James Franco inadvertently tried to pick up a teenage girl on Instagram or the football player Manti Te'o's dead girlfriend hoax? And these instances didn't even involve something as delicate as fetish. Even if an online relationship has been established, you're still meeting a virtual stranger. Use common sense and take safety precautions.

Fetish Events

Another option for compartmentalizing singles are fetish events, parties and meetups. These days, many fetish groups have introductory "munches" for newcomers. Attending live, in-person parties or events gives you the opportunity to meet like-minded fetishists. It's helpful and healing to discover that you're not alone. There's no guarantee that you'll meet the girl of your dreams but that wasn't your goal. You're looking to hook up. It's not unlike going to a sex party. The goal is to interact casually and sensually, without commitment. Fetish parties and events are fine if you're clear about this fact.

Fetish meetups are generally safe places to go. Participants are very cognizant of the need for discretion. To my knowledge, no one has ever been "outed" at a fetish event—everyone there is a fetish enthusiast and has no interest in personally humiliating anyone...unless you're into that. Depending on the kind of event, you will not only meet similarly-minded people but you might also have the opportunity to participate in a fetish scene as well. Some fantasy conventions have public play areas while others encourage private meetings in designated rooms. Parties and fetish events are first-rate outlets for people with proclivities like yours.

I recommend that you attempt to socialize only if you are single or uninvolved. It doesn't matter if you want something casual. If you're married, you're married. You don't attend social events without your partner, right? Why should a fetish event be any different? I know of too many married men who have tried this option, only to have their lives horribly disrupted. Why? Because you're going to a social event filled with all kinds of people. Even if you think you're going to casually "play," you never know how your partner will perceive the interaction.

Fetish events generally host singles or consenting married couples. If you don't fit into either category, don't go. You aren't in the market. Married people lose the right to have casual sex after they take their vows. The same is true of casual fetish play. You can't do it. It's not an option, so don't even consider it.

Go Pro

Seeing a fetish professional is a viable way to compartmentalize and still get your fetish wants met in a protected, sensible, consensual way. It's a good option for the single guy who's too busy to socialize. And it's the only realistic option for someone who's married or committed.

Many men opt to go see a professional fantasy/fetish fulfiller, more commonly known as a Dominatrix. They're women who are schooled in the practice of bondage and discipline. Though they are commonly associated with sadomasochistic type of interactions, most are experienced with all sorts of fantasies and fetishes. Even yours. Although they generally cater to people who like Dominant/submissive power exchange in a dungeon setting, many are equipped to bring cross-dressing, adult baby and spanking fantasies to life within the realm of fantasy rooms. Fetishists with specific tastes like feet, medical fantasies and smothering are usually also welcomed. A dungeon is a judgment-free zone.

Another positive about fantasy/fetish workers is the fact that there is no sex or sexual contact between you and them. Therefore, there's no risk of disease or breaching your oath of marital fidelity. These women are professionally trained in fantasy/fetish fulfillment. They are paid to listen, understand and re-enact your fantasy to the best of their ability. Many are fetishists themselves or married to fetishists. For the most part they are doing this job because they genuinely like the idea of alternative forms of sexuality. They enjoy being part of a profession that offers independence, freedom and decent pay. If your tastes lean toward dominance, you can always seek out the services of a professional submissive who will most likely work with a Domina.

When you pay a fee, you're engaging in a clean transaction. There will be no aftermath or fear of confidentiality violations. These women are there to bring your fetish to life with no strings attached. The relationship is boundaried and never goes outside the frame. This means you are guaranteed to enjoy yourself without worrying about any kind of aftermath such as miscommunications, hurt feelings or a scorned lady calling your wife.

There is also no danger of any kind of personal relationship blossoming between the two of you. A good pro never discusses her private life. She will never want to see you outside of the designated meeting spot. In short, a Dominatrix is there to provide a service, a service you require and are willing to pay for.

I know many men feel reluctant to pay for an erotic service or think that the going rate is too high. To this, I respond: "What's your relationship worth?" Let me phrase it another way: How much would you pay out in alimony or child support if your relationship crumbles because your fetish can't be fulfilled within the bounds of your marriage? Your wife obviously doesn't understand the magnitude of your fetish. She won't understand your choice of compartmentalization. Seeing a pro is therefore the only way you can protect your family and keep your marriage intact.

Even if you're single, you might still want to see a professional Dom. You've already decided to compartmentalize. Why then, waste your time and effort finding a fetish playmate? Focus on meeting your life partner and get your fetish met by someone who knows what she's doing—and is happy to do it. Think of it as treating yourself out to a sumptuous dinner at a fabulous restaurant every once in a while. Sure, you can cook at home, but this is a real treat. And after all, you deserve it!

3. You can share fetish with your partner.

We've talked a great deal about disclosure. We've weighed the pros and cons. You decided to tell and you used your communication tools. Your lady is accepting of your fetish and wants to participate. Her degree of participation isn't as important as her willingness to learn more. You'll be sharing your fetish with her for a lifetime.

Remember to take very small steps. Be supportive and complimentary each time she participates. Couples who participate in fetish together reach the apex; they are the very actualization of good fantasy enactment.

Imagine Maslow's hierarchy of needs, which is popular psychological theory. Picture the traditional Food Pyramid, but with psychological attributes instead of food groups. From top to bottom on Maslow's hierarchy are self-actualization, esteem, love/belonging, safety and physiological. Having a significant other who joins with you in fetish takes you to the top of the pyramid. You have arrived.

Your spouse's participation means that there are no more secrets. You can openly look at fetish pornography online and she'll sit beside you and watch, perhaps even comment or make suggestions. Participation means that the two of you can shop for clothing, toys or props together. Participation means that she'll be happy to have fetish nights with you and that your pleasure is her pleasure.

The Identification Outlines you created from the Fetish Checklist exercise in Chapter 7 are the blueprints for disclosure. Spoon-feed the list to your partner little by little, so she can absorb it, especially if it's long or complex. She might feel a bit insecure or inept at first. Again, be aware of the complexities of your fetish. For example, if you happen to have a casting fetish, you'll have to not only tell her what you like but you'll have to teach her how to make a cast. A casting fetish requires her to put your arm or leg in a cast made of plaster of Paris. Most women (or men) won't know how to do this. You'll have to patiently show her how. And don't expect her to be successful the first time.

The same goes for those of you with a medical fetish. That requires skill and a knowledge of hygiene and sterilization. You'll have to figure it out for yourself and then teach her how use the equipment. Like how to insert a catheter, for example, or how to administer a deep enema. Always put safety first.

The same goes for intricate bondage, cock-and-ball torture as well as nipple torture. Many fetishes require skill. That's why professional Dominatrixes actually go through a period of training. If your fetish is elaborate many of the pros now offer individual or group classes for the wives of fetishists or submissives.

Healthy incorporation is mostly about joining together. There are no more secrets. There's no more shame or embarrassment. You can talk about sexuality openly and honestly. Intimacy will grow in your relationship.

Healthy incorporation also means that you're attentive to your wife's needs. Remember that fetish is but one part of you and only a small part of your committed, multifaceted relationship. Maintain diversity in your bedroom. Indulge your fetish but remember to include the sex acts that she enjoys. Don't be selfish. Be sure that she achieves a climax in the way she likes best, whether it be with your mouth, through intercourse or with a sex toy. Be appreciative of your partner. She's accepting of you. Be accepting of her as well. Relationships are all about give and take. Make fetish about both of you.

And afterwards, be sure that you process the play. Whenever you engage in any kind of fetish play, it's crucial to talk about it. Tell her what you like and remember to ask what she enjoyed too. Remember to inquire about her feelings. Was there anything that was difficult for her? Anything she'd rather not do again? Anything she'd like to do more of?

In that vein, remember to tell her what you enjoyed. Be complimentary. Be gentle if she could stand some improvement in the execution of any specific act. Always be careful that fetish is something you brought into the relationship. She's doing this for you and to be pleasing. Appreciation and gratefulness will go a long way.

In Summary

You have come to a place of self-compassion about your fetish. You no longer feel like a freak. You understand that your fetish is a small but powerful component of your sexual makeup. You have come to the place of wanting to know how to proceed with incorporating fetish into your life. You have three options:

1) You can use your fetish as reliable masturbatory material with an air of acceptance;
2) You can participate with like-minded fetishists or professionals in a compartmentalized way, or;
3) You can incorporate fetish as part of your intimate, long-term relationship.

Only you can decide which option is best for you.

Once you have an idea of your needs, it's also necessary to break them down. Naming your fetish is only the first step. It might be the only step if your potential partner flat out refuses you. However, if you are in a relationship with a more open-minded person she will be interested in knowing more. You have to be prepared and know yourself. You can't communicate deeply about your fetish until you have an intense understanding of all its components.

And remember to disclose a little about your fetish at a time. You never want to give too much information all at once. Little by little, slow and steady. After all, you don't want to overwhelm her. By knowing yourself, you will have the ability to communicate the essentials right away. As the relationship grows, you can provide the "frills" that will make your scenes more and more satisfying. Unlike "vanilla" sex, fetish has many minutiae and actually perfects over time. Think of it as you own unique brand of fine wine and savor it as such.

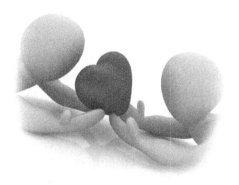

Chapter 20 – The Case Studies: Healthy Fetish Incorporation Illustrated

Healthy fetish incorporation is such a complex idea that I decided to include some real-life examples. They're based on people I've encountered in my practice as a therapist and illustrate how these people have incorporated fetish into their lives. To do so, I'll bring in case studies, some of which have been mentioned previously, but I'll dive into them more deeply here, with significant detail.

Case Study # 1 – Gary, the Spanking Fetishist

Gary is an adult male who enjoys spanking. He's painstakingly researched the subject and has had innumerable therapy sessions with me. He's had the spanking fetish as far back as he can remember. From the moment he hit puberty, he sought out ways to get this fetish in his life. Along the way, Gary's journey took some dysfunctional turns. He'd engage in spanking talk with young mothers who discipline their children that way. He'd try to get housekeepers to discipline him for keeping his house dirty. He'd even seduce his boss to discipline him at the office. All very disordered ways to get his spanking fetish into his life. What's wrong with his behavior?

Gary's most glaring hallmark of inappropriateness was engaging in fetish play with non-consenting adults. The young mothers never had a clue that Gary was getting titillated during their casual chats about spanking. The housekeepers were there to clean, not spank a grown man. And the most dangerous act of all was disclosing his predilections in the workplace. Gary is lucky his behavior didn't get him fired or arrested. Very lucky. He and I have done extensive work together and he's come very far.

Understanding and acceptance were key components to Gary's case. He came from a chaotic home. His parents fought constantly, and as a result Gary soothed himself with masturbation and thoughts of spanking. As an adult, Gary found that he particularly needed to have some kind of spanking talk in order to "self soothe" and relieve his stress. Eventually, he came to a place where he understood the background of his fetish, how it served him growing up and how it clearly wasn't a good idea to engage in spanking talk with non-consensual adults.

Gary also came to realize that he did enjoy talking about spanking and actualizing it with females who were both on the giving and receiving end. He was able to have his desires met by seeing professionals who understood the fetish of spanking. This was great because he could have his spanking desires satisfied by women who consensually wanted to engage with him. Often called Dominatrixes, these women choose to be sex workers who specialize in fulfilling the fantasies of adult fetishists. Gary sought out professionals who understood his desire to talk about spanking and then receive one in the form of a pre-planned role-play. Although Gary learned how to satisfy his spanking needs, he still wasn't satisfied.

Gary came to the slow realization that he wanted to have spanking incorporated into his adult life. He was still single when we started working together so he tried out a variety of ways to approach women with his fetish. He'd date women from Internet dating sites, women he met at various social gatherings and also tried dating women he found online on fetish social networking sites. The more Gary dated, the more he became comfortable talking about his fetish and communicating his cravings.

Though Gary liked to both give and receive spankings, he reached the conclusion that he'd be most happy with a woman who would give him a spanking. He realized that giving a spanking himself was nice but not essential for his long-term satisfaction. He also understood that talking about spanking was probably the thing he liked most about his fetish. He enjoyed hearing words related to spanking, key phrases and certain aspects of spanking that could occur in real life (these would be fantasy based, of course).

As time progressed, Gary finally, met the woman he married through an introduction from a colleague. Rita wasn't a spanking fetishist but she was open-minded and very much in love with Gary. She thought his spanking predilections a little strange but not off-putting. Gary was able to communicate what he wanted to Rita and she was happy to please the guy she loved. In turn, Gary was an attentive, supportive partner and ready to meet her every emotional need.

Gary was able to incorporate his spanking fetish in a healthy way. It took quite some time but eventually he realized that his approach of engaging with non-consensual women wasn't helpful in any way. He got his compulsive behaviors under control largely by accepting that his fetish was real, okay and here to stay. Then he figured out exactly what he wanted by allowing himself to engage with professional women who were experienced with spanking and happy to satisfy his spanking fantasies in a proficient manner where safe boundaries were established.

Finally, Gary made the decision that he wanted to play in a standard type of committed relationship. Because he was already comfortable with his fetish, he was able to articulate his wishes in a way that was inviting and enticing to the women he dated. Finally, he chose a woman who was compatible with him on every level. Rita had similar values and principles in life as well as parallel spiritual beliefs. They also enjoyed many of the same bedroom activities. His bride is happy to spank him physically and engage in spanking verbiage. She's even open to taking Gary to a Spanking Specialist to celebrate special occasions.

Did Gary hit the fetish jackpot or was he ready to have a well-rounded relationship that allowed for fetish play in addition to all the key elements of a well-balanced relationship? Whatever the response, Gary is in a good place because he approached his fetish in an adult, comprehensive way.

Case Study # 2 – Brian, the Diaper Fetishist

Brian likes to dress in diapers. (I briefly mentioned him in Chapter 11.) Brian doesn't want to be "babied," dominated or humiliated. He simply likes the feel of wearing diapers to bed. Imagine how difficult this could be for a married guy. He worried, 'How am I going to share this with my wife? It's so embarrassing. I can't do it.'

Brian ultimately found a very creative way of getting what he wanted. For years he lied and told his wife he was incontinent. She thought he simply had to wear diapers for medical reasons. She never questioned it. There was never an issue until one day, she caught Brian wearing a diaper and masturbating to infantilism pornography. Obviously his wife was shocked and he was mortified. That's when Brian came to see me.

When we first began counseling, Brian had no clue about the nature of fetish. All he was aware of was that he wanted to wear diapers, the satisfaction he received from wearing them and that diapers was a lifelong habit. Of course, he knew that others shared his interest but he was very unaware about the implications of his fetish.

Our first number of meetings were spent on education, understanding fetish in general, eventually learning more about the infantilism fetish and the possible meanings attached to the fetish for Brian. In his case, we connected some truths about very real neglect in his early days. Brian's parents were both very busy people deeply engaged in their careers. As a result, Brian was often left with a variety of caretakers which led to the early stages of anxiety. It makes sense that Brian probably developed some kind of feelings of security when his diaper was being changed. At that moment, someone was taking care of him and he wasn't being ignored. In fact, he was receiving wonderful attention, perhaps even was cooed to and tickled.

Discovering the "why" helped Brian come to a place of understanding about his fetish. Talking about and exploring his needs also helped him feel more accepting and comfortable with his yen to be diapered. But how was he going to explain this yearning to his wife Gloria, who was seething at his deceit and totally confused?

Obviously, this was a big one. The more Brian explored, he identified the fact that his wish was to wear diapers. His wish was not to be deceitful. In fact, in many ways it was a relief that his wife found out. He hated the deception and Gloria's concern about incontinence. Ironically, Brian rarely even urinated in the diaper. His wish was all about the tactile comfort of diaper-wearing. He simply liked the fabric and feel of the diaper against his skin.

Once Brian was comfortable and came to embrace self-compassion, he was able to communicate with Gloria in a kind, gentle voice. First, he apologized for lying. He disclosed his fetish needs and the embarrassment and shame that came along with them. He explained how he wanted to tell Gloria but just didn't have the courage. He also told her that he made the decision he wanted to continue to wear diapers. He explained that this was a craving which wouldn't go away and he didn't want to make a promise that he couldn't' keep. In other words, if Brian told Gloria he wouldn't wear diapers any more, chances were good he'd find another way to have his needs met in secret. And he didn't want to do that.

Because Brian was comfortable with is fetish, he was able to communicate in a way that made Gloria comfortable, too. She was actually happy to know that her husband didn't have a physical disorder as she imagined and that his fetish (unlike the serious prostate issues she feared!) was something that was relatively easy to control. All she had to do was add adult diapers to her shopping list.

The best part about all of this was that Brian's wife was a good lady who wanted to join with her husband in his fetish. Gloria actually went online and looked at some of his favorite infantile sites. Together, they discovered ways to incorporate diapering into sensual bedroom play. Brian never had the opportunity to do this with anyone before and he fell in love with

Gloria all over again. They are both living happily ever after in a guilt-free relationship. The benefits of disclosure led to healthy incorporation of fetish. Brian wished he'd had the courage to tell his wife before, but better late than never!

Case Study # 3 – Calvin, the Male Submissive

Calvin is a submissive male. He's been that way all his life. As the youngest of five children, all of Calvin's siblings are girls. So, you can safely surmise that catering to females is something that comes naturally to him. Growing up, Calvin's sisters would not only coddle him but they would often play with him in an aggressive manner. They would order him about, make him do their chores and take turns "mothering" him.

Their own mother was a busy lady so she depended on her girls to look after themselves—and their baby brother. She delegated the task of taking care of Calvin, her last born (probably unplanned child or her last-ditch attempt to have a son) to her daughters. Their dad was also very much out of the picture since he had a job that required lots of travel. It seemed that Calvin's parents had a distant but workable relationship. They probably stayed together because most of the time they were apart.

Calvin's sisters played an integral role in his development. He really identified with the idea of being the baby and in a large part, he played the role of his sisters' plaything. They would often gang up on him in a humorous manner. Calvin remembers sometimes being the butt of their teasing. They'd play games where he was the villain and was tied up for questioning. Every now and again, they would dress him in their feminine clothes. Calvin was a good-natured boy and probably liked the attention. But whatever the case, he never rebelled or protested. He embraced his role of baby brother.

It makes sense, then, that Calvin would identify with being a submissive male. Not that every male who has many older female siblings, turns to D/s activities to derive sexual pleasure, but Calvin did. Calvin enjoys many aspects of Dominant/submissive play. He likes the idea of a Dominant female dressed in leather, especially thigh boots. He loves heavy bondage in conjunction with nipple torture, flogging and some mild forms of humiliation. In fact, in Calvin's fantasy scenarios, there's nothing he wouldn't do for his Goddess.

Early on, Calvin suspected he had these predilections but kept them to himself. He remembers liking certain strong female characters like Catwoman and Elvira. Even comic-book drawings of tough females like Storm, from the Fantastic Four, turned him on the same way most of his friends were aroused by Playboy centerfolds. But most of the time, he kept these images to himself and pulled them out of his head and into his consciousness when he was alone masturbating. He reasoned that no one had to know and that he'd go to the grave with his secret.

Calvin eventually married and had daughters of his own. He was the doting husband and father—always giving, never taking. Calvin worked hard and provided well for his family. On the surface, he appeared to be the guy who had it all yet somewhere deep down he knew there was something missing.

This missing piece became apparent to Calvin while surfing on the Internet one day. When he happened on a site dedicated to his fetish, he describes it like being "as if I had come home." Of course, Calvin didn't just stumble upon these websites by accident, but Calvin told himself that he did. Somehow or other, he typed in a key word or phrase that led him to the place he wanted to go.

Calvin was hooked. After that, he spent hours online masturbating. He was like a bird let out of a very tiny cage. He spent hours online visiting every website devoted to his fetish that he could find. Calvin absorbed a lifetime of fantasy into the course of a six-month "cramfest" online. He told his wife Liz that he was involved in a research project for work, but of course, the only truthful thing about his explanation was word "research." He was researching his fetish to death!

Calvin was clueless, lost and didn't know how to approach Liz about his fetish. His fear was that she'd ridicule him, degrade him and abandon him. And Calvin wasn't far off in his thinking. It's no surprise that Calvin had chosen a wife that had some of the qualities of his beloved sisters—Liz was strong-minded and sometimes domineering. This was reflected in the way she dealt with his fetish—which wasn't good.

And neither was the way Calvin revealed his fetish to her. One day, he couldn't take the pressure of holding his fetish inside anymore. He simply blurted out his passion to Liz and came clean about the fact that some of the mysterious credit card charges on their AmEx were in fact his. Understandably, Liz was extremely angry. He feared that she'd be upset but he had no idea about how upset. Basically, Liz told him to ditch his fetish or leave their 15-year relationship. That's when Calvin came to me. Together, Calvin and I went through the steps in my program laboriously. He had to learn about fetish and come to place of self-acceptance and understanding. This took months, as we had to dig deep and figure out the old messages he received from his childhood.

The more Calvin talked about his sexual predilections, the more he wanted to have a real-time experience. Since Liz was so unwilling to have anything to do with his fetish, Calvin chose to go to a qualified, experienced, professional Dominatrix who was willing to take it slow with a newbie. Before he went to his session, Calvin and I had explored the pros and cons of his decision. Calvin felt he owed it to himself to have this very important real-time enactment of his fantasies.

As you might have guessed, Calvin loved his first experience enacting his fetish. Though the Dominatrix started out slowly, his level of excitement was so high, and his endorphins flowed so greatly that he never registered pain when she whipped him. Only sublime pleasure.

Calvin decided that he definitely wanted to incorporate his D/s desires into his life. His preference was to do this with his wife. Though their children were just about grown (three out of four were college graduates), he still wanted to keep his family intact. However, the more he talked, explored and thought about his fetish, the more he realized that he wanted to have it in his life on some level.

Calvin saw his fetish as a passion, a passion that had lay dormant for decades. He decided that he wanted to treat this fetish like a beloved hobby. As a result, Calvin started to cut back on his online adult website viewing and treated himself to a professional Dominatrix session only on special occasions. His anxiety level was down because he knew that Doms were readily available, and so was the adult material he liked to look at. The more Calvin figured out what he liked, the more confident he felt in his ability to control and manage his fetish. The final challenge was how to tell Liz that he wouldn't comply with her wishes to end it.

Liz had been pretty patient. She took comfort in the fact that Calvin was in therapy and felt certain that one day, he'd come to his senses. When they finally had the discussion about his fetish in my office, Liz was pretty horrified, angry and disappointed that he'd decided to go against her wishes. She couldn't understand that his fetish predated his relationship with her—and that it would be there forever. And this was exactly the problem. Calvin was always succumbing to Liz's wishes, just as he had with his sisters. At this point, Calvin was totally accepting of his fetish and with that came a huge boost in his self-esteem.

The three of us had many conjoint sessions together. I worked with Liz according to the plan I laid out in Sex, Fetish and Him. However, one can't change their thinking unless they're willing. And Calvin's wife wasn't. Instead, she was rigid and resolute in her original proclamation: "Leave the fetish or leave the marriage."

In the end, Calvin chose to leave his marriage. He left honorably, responsibly and maintains a good relationship with his grown children. He provides financial support in the way of alimony to his ex-wife and is always available in times of emergency. But Calvin also has his self-respect and dignity intact. Ironically, now that he's single, Calvin spends very little time online and has yet to see a professional Dominatrix. He's beginning to date women his own age who are compatible with him spiritually, educationally and professionally.

Newly-divorced, Calvin is allowing himself the time to enjoy the company of many women. When he finds the woman he plans to become intimate with, he expects to reveal his fetish details before heading to the bedroom. He's very confident that his knowledge and expertise will convey the fact to her that his fetish is a source of pleasure and he's inviting her in to join in the fun. He has a good, positive mindset and is certain that if she's the right woman, she'll want to make him happy. Meanwhile, he continues to be desirable dating material that many women are currently enjoying.

Case Study # 4 – Amir, the Macrophiliac

You briefly met Amir in Chapter 15. He came to me with help for his fetish, which is coined "macrophilia." It's a fancy word for a simple fetish that's nearly impossible to attain. Amir likes the idea of having sex with women who are very big. Almost giantesses. To him, it's the ultimate form of domination. Amir likes to view himself as a small object at the feet of a very, very large Amazonian female. The taller, the better. He also likes the idea of a woman who's muscular. The height difference makes him want to melt, he says.

Amir remembers thinking about this fetish ever since he was a young boy. Maybe it has something to do with his Middle Eastern background and growing up in a war-torn country, but Amir took solace in the idea of a big woman taking care of him. Of course, this idea of creating a female as a conqueror of the male totally goes against his culture. This is one of the reasons Amir kept the fantasy to himself…until his company transferred him to Los Angeles.

Now Amir happily found himself in the Mecca of a free-thinking culture but still, it wasn't easy for him to date. Notwithstanding the language barrier and being a foreigner in a strange new world, Amir wanted to date women who stand at seven feet high. Well, that's a tall order (no pun intended) for anyone! Where would he find a towering, muscular honey to be the life partner of a five-foot five-inch tall Arabic guy?

In our therapy sessions, Amir and I talked about this endlessly and he didn't want to deviate from his fantasy. He even sought out professional Dominatrixes who billed themselves as "tall." And alas, they were tall but never tall enough. Amir and I discussed the possibility of his dating and eventually doing some role play with a "vanilla" love interest but that didn't satisfy Amir either.

Finally, we decided that Amir would have to come to the realization that no girl could reasonably meet his needs. His fetish was very fantasy-based, and as a result, it would have to stay in Fantasyland. With that understanding, Amir looked to the Internet as a vehicle to incorporate his fetish in a healthy way. It turns out that there are actually websites devoted to macrophilia media. Amir discovered manipulated photographs, cartoons and fantasy fiction stories that specifically catered to his fetish. He allowed himself to browse and enjoy.

Once Amir relaxed, he let his mind explore other possibilities. He looked into the related trampling fetish, where a woman walks on a man's chest. He also returned to the Bondage Parlor and had a satisfying experience with a woman who was tall, but not freakishly so. With my guidance, Amir learned compromise as a way to incorporate fetish into his life in a healthy way.

Case Study # 5 – Clay, the Foot Fetishist

Clay has a simple foot fetish with a twist. He enjoys worshipping a bare female foot but only if the soles are very rough. A ballerina or an avid hiker might be a perfect match for him but so far he hasn't found a woman with soles tough enough to his liking.

In our therapy sessions, Clay and I went over and over the ways he could possibly get his partners' feet to be rough enough for his fantasies. However, each time, he found a flaw in my plan. He claimed that he tried to roughen up his partners' feet by having the women walk barefoot on the beach but the quality of the coarseness was never quite right and not what he was after. Clay tried to discount his tactile prerequisite for roughness but that never worked out either.

It probably didn't take you too long to figure out that Clay is fussy. He's no different from the kind of person who finds something wrong with every woman he dates. Clay is still convinced he will find the woman with "perfect rough soles."

But never forget, this is Clay's fetish and ultimately, his choice. He made a decision that feet were his priority. Clay is okay with this decision that will probably sentence him to a lifetime of frustration—and guaranteed bachelorhood. Still, it's his choice so it has to be respected. Maybe someday, he'll reach a place of happy compromise like Amir did, but I don't think it will be any time soon. Just as long as Clay is fine with this and it doesn't cause him too much anguish, it's not a bad place to be.

The Heathy Incorporation Lifestyle

When you've made the decision to incorporate your fetish into your relationship in a healthy manner, there are a number of things to remember:

1. Choose Wisely

Be thoughtful about choosing the right person for you. Remember that sexual compatibility is only one of many categories to consider in a life partner. Dating allows you to get to know someone. If you're in your 20s or 30s and looking for a life partner, you're not only seeking someone you want to spend the rest of your life with but many times, you are also looking for the mother of your children. You must ask yourself important questions like, Is she trustworthy? Does she have your back? Do you enjoy your time with her both in and out of the bedroom? Does she laugh at your jokes? Do you feel good in her presence?

Most notably, do you two truly, deeply love each other? When I say "love," I'm talking about unconditional acceptance. This means she loves you for who you are. She doesn't want to change you. She will be supportive of your goals, but in the end, she will be there for you no matter what. She loves you as you are and doesn't see you as a diamond in the rough or a house requiring extensive renovation.

If your woman truly loves you, she will want to do the things that make you happy. This means she will want to engage with you in your fetish. Not necessarily because the act, costume or object is her fantasy but because she gets pleasure in pleasing you.

But this doesn't mean she's a doormat either! You will also derive a great deal of pleasure in pleasing her. Love, with a side order of fetish, is a two-way street and is all about compromise. Even if she's not a giantess she'd be more than happy to play the role of an Amazonian woman for you. Even if she was brought up to think that men must be the aggressor, she will welcome the idea of switching roles.

In general, she's the type of gal who will bring over a sack of potatoes from the grocery store just because you texted and asked her to make the stop. She will do it because you asked and won't question your motive. She loves you and wants to do what it takes to be with you—and you'd do the same for her.

You won't find her spending too much time at the bar, the gym or online. She's the one doing volunteer work for handicapped kids or giving her time at the nursing home. She's beautiful both inside and out.

2. Look No Further Than Your Partner

You made your choice years ago. You have a wife and hopefully, she's a good one. You've released your shame and have come to a place of self-acceptance. You really understand your fetish now and you feel confident in your ability to communicate. While doing this soul-searching you've decided that your preference is to participate with your wife. Good for you. Now it's time to get a plan in place.

Remember to never rush into introducing your fetish to your partner. It might have taken you a long time to reveal your secret in the right way. If you take steps to enact your fetish slowly and mindfully, your experience will be that much greater. Don't forget that she needs to be introduced to your fetish as though it's a good friend of yours from the past whom she's never met. (In a sense, it is.) If this new friend is here to stay and you want her to spend time with them, easy does it. She has to gradually acclimate to this friend. You wouldn't want to have your friend over for dinner every night, would you? Probably not. Maybe for an introductory cup of coffee one day and dinner another. See what I mean? Nobody wants anything thrust upon them suddenly, especially something as big a deal as a fetish.

Follow steps outlined in this book to help guide you. Start with a general discussion about fetish. Ask her what she knows about the subject and then share your knowledge with her. Unless she asks specially, you don't have to disclose all of the intimate details of your fetish right away. Do it slowly but surely. Try to incorporate some aspect of the fetish during foreplay. For example, if you're a foot fetishist, you can spend more time wor-shipping her feet. It's all about being deliberate and patient.

Once she's comfortable, you can start to communicate more. During this early phase, be super-attentive to her. The nicer you are to her, the nicer she'll be to you. Make sure that her needs are being met. This means her emotional as well as her sexual needs. Spend extra time listening to her talk about her day. Take a real

Fetish and You

interest in the family. Be an ideal husband and you will have an appreciative wife who is more receptive about learning about your "quirk."

Always remember to have a sense of humor about your fetish. Try to put yourself in her shoes as you talk. Remember that she'll be shocked at first but she will eventually (hopefully!) follow your lead. If you present as confident, she'll feel comfortable with the topic. Let her ask questions. Share some benign images that illustrate aspects of the fetish. Take it slow. Be honest and vulnerable.

Remember, this is the woman you chose to spend your life with. She loves you and wants you to feel good. When the time is right, you might also have her read relevant chapters from my book *Sex, Fetish and Him*. Better yet, read it together. Answer the questions that pertain to your fetish and about fetish in general. If she's the right woman, she'll eventually understand and will join with you on your fetish journey.

3. Time to Move On

So, what if you didn't choose so wisely? What if you tried your best to engage your partner and she is oppositional to your desires? Of course, the decision to leave a marriage is a difficult one to make and should only be taken as a last resort after all other options have been exhausted.

In my experience, it's almost never the fetish itself that breaks up a couple; it's the rejection and conditional love that tears couples apart. If you thought she would be open to your fetish and she isn't, please keep trying. This might be the perfect time to have her read the first few chapters of *Sex, Fetish and Him*. Especially the chapter that focuses on the fetish mindset, which is called "Understanding Offbeat Sexuality."

Remember it wasn't so long ago that you felt uncomfortable about being a fetishist. She must have some time to digest and retrain her brain. She has to consider the idea that "out-of-the-box" sexuality isn't wrong or perverse. It's simply different. Fetish doesn't define you. Fetish is only one small aspect of the husband she has adored up until now.

But maybe your wife hasn't been as adoring as you think. Perhaps the disclosure of your fetish is the excuse she was looking for to bail out of the relationship. If so, you'll know it. Calvin didn't leave his marriage because his wife rejected his interest in BDSM. He left because his wife was rejecting of him. That's a big difference. You'll know it if you see it.

4. Getting Real with Your Fetish

If you have distinctive tastes, you might have to redefine them. Ask yourself, "Does my partner have to actively engage in my fetish? Will I ever find someone who fits the bill?"

Amir finally came to see that he could never find a woman who is tall enough and large enough to fit his fantasy. Once he made that realization, his anxiety about never finding that "perfect giantess" waned and it allowed him to relax and enjoy his fetish online. By taking the pressure off of himself, he allowed his brain to be more receptive to other fantasies that were similar but more plausible than macrophilia.

Hence, Amir allowed himself to be open to trampling, which is something that virtually any woman can do. All trampling requires is for him to lie flat on his back and have his partner step on him with her bare feet. Amir loves trampling now. And guess what? When Amir is flat on his back, his female partners appear very, very tall to him. And again, this fantasy is extremely easy. To date, no partner has refused him. Amir is very confident that he will find his life partner within the next couple of years.

So, compromise is sometimes essential. What will your woman do and what would be absurd to ask someone to do? Toilet slavery is generally pretty much a "no, no" for most women, especially anything to do with feces. However, your wife might be willing to talk "potty talk" with you during some masturbatory play.

RCR (Relax, Come, Relax) is a concept I mentioned back in Chapter 14 and also discuss in *Sex, Fetish and Him*. I advise women who don't want to physically participate in a fetish to talk about the fetish with their man. With RCR, the man can pleasure himself or his partner can masturbate him while supplying some sexy, fetish talk. Then, he gets close to climax, she stops, he relaxes and she starts up again. (You can also try doing this to her!) It's a pleasurable exercise which I bet will satisfy your fetish jones. Although talk is easy (and cheap), it can also be very gratifying and bring you both closer together.

Again, it's imperative to choose the woman who is open to fetish and wants to join in it with you. There are so many ways to participate in a fetish—and not just physically. The beauty of it is that you can explore each of them together.

5. Forget About It

If you're like Clay, you're probably destined to be alone. You should stop using your fetish as the excuse for your solitary state. Embrace the idea that you have chosen to shut people out of your fetish because you can never find the "perfect" partner. Ultimately, your preference is to stay single. And if this is the case, just accept the idea and stop wasting everyone's time by searching for a fetish partner who will never be "right" in your estimation.

However if you ultimately want to change, you have to do the work. Start thinking about compromise and be empathetic to others. Seek out some counseling and figure out your fears about intimacy. I'm sure you are a good guy and want more than a solitary life of you and your fetish object.

In Summary

As you can see from the case studies, people choose to incorporate fetish in a variety of ways. Only you can decide which is best for you. Only you know what life situation you're faced with. While fetish fulfillment will not be your biggest priority if you have a wife and children, fetish still must be given a place in your life. Finding room for your fetish is the basic goal of healthy incorporation. I'm confident you can figure out something, no matter the situation or how impossible it may seem. Remember to consider others but also remember that you are important, too. Healthy balance is what you want to achieve here.

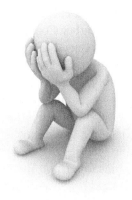

Chapter 21 - Managing Your Fetish

I admit, it's difficult to manage your fetish when it seems to be everywhere. Here are a few examples of fetish-management challenges—and solutions:

Ryan is a young college student who's having difficulty with his foot fetish. He loves bare feet the way many men love breasts. He seeks my help during springtime in Los Angeles when the weather is warm and girls are switching from boots to summer shoes. During lectures, Ryan's surrounded by female classmates wearing open-toed shoes and sandals. Understandably, he's having a tough time concentrating on his schoolwork. "To me, it's the equivalent of sitting in a roomful of topless dancers," he explains. "It's way too distracting." Ryan requested help controlling his raging hormones.

Larry is in his mid-40s and has a leather fetish. He gets very turned-on seeing women dressed in long leather coats and boots. Is it any wonder? Larry hails from Canada and has many memories of his mother's friends coming to visit bundled in their plush leather jackets. As a boy, it was his job to help Mom's friends remove their coats and hang them up. Something internally happened during this time which Larry's brain registered as arousal. As a result, he now has a fetish for these garments. Larry still resides in Canada and lucky for him, leather coats never go out of style. But each winter he faces a major dilemma—how to live in Leather Coat Heaven and still function in his daily life. Larry clearly needs help managing his impulses.

Richard is in his 30s and is a nonsmoker. Yet, he has a fetish for women who smoke long, slender cigarettes. He often goes outside to watch his coworkers blissfully inhaling. Every now and again, there's one or two who smoke his brand of choice. When that happens, Richard's inclination is to head straight for the bathroom and masturbate. He knows it's inappropriate behavior for the workplace and tries to refrain. But once or twice, he's had to leave work early. Richard is concerned that his feelings may escalate to the point that he'll do something he regrets.

As a fetishist, you may find yourself encountering real-life situations like Ryan, Larry and Richard that trigger arousal responses. At a moment's notice, you find yourself getting sexually excited. This can happen in the supermarket, mall or even at church. A visual image, verbal phrase or a facial expression can set your heart—and your pants— on fire without warning. The timing is inappropriate yet the craving is there, loud and clear. Sometimes it's really difficult to handle.

It's one thing to accept yourself and be guilt-free. But it's quite another thing to live in a world where temptation lies at every corner. It's like an alcoholic being let loose in a bar. Or a diabetic being locked in an ice cream truck. The urge to satisfy your impulse is overwhelming. Intellectually you know the difference between right and wrong, appropriate verses inappropriate behavior. But during these unexpected fetish moments, you feel weak with longing. It's very easy to want to give into your impulses. You want to seize the moment so badly, but you don't. The risk is too high and the repercussions would be too serious.

It may feel like no one would understand this dilemma. It may feel as though life has dealt you an impossibly difficult hand of cards. You feel weird enough about your fetish without having to wrestle with this level of temptation. Acting out in public is the very last thing you want to do. But that moment, you can't help but think about how exciting it would be to act spontaneously. To touch, smell and embrace the desired object, body part or material.

Ryan expressed it best when he said to me, "Life is so unfair. College is hard enough. It's important that I concentrate but I can't because bare feet are all around me. The toes are adorned with the red polish I love. It kills me. Other guys don't have this problem because they're turned-on by body parts that are covered up."

And that's true. You can probably empathize with Ryan because you've been there, too. Ryan was smart enough to get some help before he let his feelings overtake his logic. But sometimes the impulses win out. When they do, you will be entering dangerous territory like some fetishists I've treated. Like Barry, for example.

When Barry was a college student, he found a way to indulge his spanking fetish. He'd get out the phone book and randomly call up women. He pretended he was doing a research paper on the pros and cons of spanking. He'd interview unsuspecting mothers over the telephone and ask them all sorts of questions about spanking. Two years later, he grew bolder and would actually ask women to show him what a real spanking felt like. Many actually complied.

Tim likes silk pantyhose. He often corners women at the mall to talk to them about their legwear. He asks them questions about the material, brand name and where to get them, all under the guise of pretending to be buying them for his wife. Tim will also browse lingerie shops to chat up the salesladies about pantyhose. He'll talk for as long as they let him. Sometimes he makes a purchase but often he doesn't.

Jerome loves to attend garage sales. As a shoe fetishist, he will rummage through the high heels. He enjoys quizzing the sellers about the various pairs of shoes they're selling. He asks things like, "Where did you buy them? For what occasion? How long have you had them?" Jerome can go on like this for hours. Finally, he'll make a purchase, generally leaving with a bagful of heels At this point, Jerome is deep into his fetish zone. He's almost unaware of everything except his growing penis. He gets into his car and masturbates fast, before anyone can see. To date, he hasn't been caught but there's always a first time. He's walking on thin ice.

Barry, Tim and Jerome are engaging in disordered fetish behavior. Why is it disordered? Because the interactions are all non-consensual. All the women were clueless to the fact that they were engaging with a fetishist. They had no idea that their words were being interpreted as sexual, masturbatory material or that they were being manipulated for someone's prurient interests. Can you see what's wrong with this? While it's true that the ladies never knew what was going on, imagine that they did. I bet they'd consider themselves violated and being used.

Often, fetishists who engage with non-consenting people get caught. The victims feel traumatized. They describe it as being similar to rape. That's because they weren't aware of what was going on. They think the fetishist took advantage of them. Some victims will be silent but many will speak out. Imagine the repercussions. Reputations could be damaged. Careers could be ruined. Worst of all, legal charges could be filed. All because a fetishist couldn't keep his fantasies in check. I hope you read these words with trepidation and that this never happens to you.

If you feel tempted or have thoughts about acting out non-consensually, you must work on managing your impulse control. You might even require professional help with your fetish management. If you absolutely can't do it on your own, get some guidance from an addiction therapist or 12-Step Program.

Remember, though, that many therapists and some programs aren't always going to be fetish-friendly. Unfortunately, many in my field are still pretty uniformed about fetish. Still, you need help. But always be aware of this: You're seeking help not because you have a fetish, but because you're out of control. It's why alcoholics go to AA. Eventually they find that one drink turns into too many. They don't want to drink a lot but the liquor is more powerful than their intellect.

It's not that the alcohol is inherently wrong, it's that the individual can't manage his drinking. While I'm aware of the fact that people with a drinking problem are told that they can never drink again, I'm not suggesting that disordered fetishists have to give up their fetish thoughts. While nobody must have liquor, you do need to have sexuality in your life. You just have to learn how to embrace your fetish in a way that is a way that can fit into your lifestyle with your partner or consenting adults.

If you know that you're letting your inclinations get the better of you, take pause. Think of the consequences of your behavior. If you honestly can't control yourself, then you must admit that you have a problem and seek out help as an addict or an alcoholic. Don't, however, seek help because you have a sexual fetish.

Many in the psychological community will tell you that fetish is an addiction. But I don't believe this is true. A fetish can be an addiction if you let it get the best of you, but it doesn't always have to be an addiction. And by "getting the best of you," I mean that you buy into the idea that you have no control because the fetish is all around you. If you feel that you have no choice but to run to the nearest bathroom and masturbate when confronted with one of your fetish triggers in your day-to-day life, remember that you do have a choice, and the choice is yours.

When you're in a public place, abide by the common standards of etiquette. You can glance but you can't stare. You can look but you can't touch. Let's be frank— you have to behave like a human being, not an animal. How is that different from anyone else and their desires?

You truly aren't that different than anyone else. Don't buy into the nonsense that you have something wrong with you. Don't listen to those who tell you it's imperative for you to give up your fetish. As much as many of you might want to rid yourself of your fetish, it's impossible. It can't happen because this is the way you're wired. No matter how much you'd like to take a pill and have your fetish disappear, it won't happen. Your fetish may lay dormant for a few years but it always comes back. Trust me, I've worked with hundreds of people who tried not to think about their fetish but it always reared its lovely head again. Why? Because the fetish is deeply ingrained and ultimately, we're all sexual creatures. Fetish is merely the way you express your sexuality.

The fact that you're a fetishist, doesn't mean you can't have self-control; it's simply being sexually appropriate. The more you feel okay about your fetish, the more peaceful you'll feel. With peace comes a sense of well-being. Reducing stress will allow you to enjoy your fetish moments. You won't have a need to compulsively self-soothe. You can learn to be sexual at the proper time and place. All adults do this. You certainly can, too.

Let's Talk about Management

I can't help but think of the old Henny Youngman joke. A man goes to the doctor because his arm hurts when he raises it. The patient says, "Doctor, it hurts when I do this." And the doctor tells him, "Then don't do that!"

Managing fetish doesn't have to be complicated. It's pretty simple. Just use common sense. Ryan simply has to keep his eyes on the professor, not on the floor. In our work together, Ryan and I explored his way of thinking and the messages he was giving himself. It turns out that he bought into the idea that his fetish was his downfall. He believed that without his fetish, he would have no problems with school work. That wasn't necessarily the case. There were other issues at hand beside his foot fetish. He also had to study more and concentrate more! When we investigated the validity of his thinking, Ryan finally realized that he was the one in control, not his foot fetish. Once he changed his thinking, Ryan found his grades and attentiveness improved.

Barry needed a safe place to talk. Random strangers were not the answer. He first had to educate himself about fetish and understand that it was fine to engage in spanking play with other consenting adults. Finally, it was imperative for Barry to get in touch with the grave consequences of his actions. While he initially thought it was all right to converse with unsuspecting mothers over the phone, he never realized how profoundly dishonest he was being.

The calls were not about research; they were about sex since spanking was his fetish. Therefore, these were phone sex calls that Barry was getting for free. Not cool and not fair to anyone. The same thing goes for visiting strangers' houses under the false pretenses of doing spanking research. This was extremely risky behavior which could have put Barry in the hospital, in jail or worse. It was definitely not worth taking the chance. But once Barry understood the nature of his fetish, he was able to incorporate it into his life in a healthy manner.

Jerome also needed the help that you're getting with this book. He didn't understand his fetish and how profoundly it impacted his life. He also never considered the fact that his communication with unsuspecting strangers was inappropriate. Once Jerome received counseling from me, he understood his cravings.

Jerome is currently in the process of talking to his wife about his pantyhose fetish. There was some truth in his telling women that he was buying the pantyhose for his partner but in truth, his wife had no clue why he was doing so. Deep down, he actually wanted to see her wearing them and he's finally mustered the courage to tell her.

Disordered behavior largely comes from misinformation, untruths and falsehoods about sex. Society's rigid standards and beliefs often trigger feelings of unworthiness. When we feel that we are "less than" or have something to hide, we act inappropriately. We also feel we must be secretive and act improperly in order to get our needs met.

At this point, you know better. You know what fetish is all about. You're aware of your outlets. You know the difference between consenting adults and non-consenting adults. And that's really the key. Any time you engage with a person who isn't aware of what you're doing, she's non-consenting. Therefore, professionals or other fetishists are fair game because they are aware of your fetish and they are willingly participating.

Ultimately, you want to be in control of your fetish. You do not want your fetish to control you. You are the captain of your ship. You don't have to be caught up by your fetish. You can choose to stay in control. You're the same as everybody else. And all of us have to learn how to control our sexual urges. It's what separates us from our cousins, the apes.

The real difference for you as a fetishist is the fact that you're turned-on by something unique. That's all. Everything else is the same — with one happy exception. You have something that will reliably arouse for the rest of your life. You will not lose your sex drive at age 50, 60 or beyond. Fetish is that powerful. You'll be happily titillated for the rest of your days. Just don't abuse your sexual gift. Use it wisely with other consensual adults and you'll be fine.

How to Behave

My suggestion about how to behave properly is normalization. Sexual triggers exist all around us. Does the foot fetishist really have it any worse than the breast or butt man? Bathing suits, summer clothing and alluring evening wear all accentuate parts of the female body which are desirous to most men. However, as intelligent humans, we know how to regulate our urges and act out with a consensual partner at appropriate times. The sexy stimuli are just that. The female anatomy is sexually objectified even for the straightest of men. Eyeing the special body parts produce pleasant sensations that can be appreciated in the moment and fantasized about later. It's really no different for the fetishist. I promise.

Yes, it's true that fetishes are very strong. The triggers may be more intense than what most people experience. Sexual urges are instinctual. We are no different than animals. And guess what sets us apart from the common, every day mammal? Our intelligence, superego and the ability to reason. We all know how to behave appropriately. So, the foot fetishist has the same choice as the breast or butt man. Don't ogle. Don't make your intentions known. You can gaze but don't gawk. And most of all, keep your mind focused at the task at hand.

We all have the ability to control ourselves. And that includes you. You have the capability to find a bathroom before urinating in your pants, correct? You can say no to that second piece of pie instead of giving in, right? You also understand the virtues of delayed gratification. You have the ability to exercise restraint and control.

So yes, you might be tempted when you find yourself in a fetishist environment but honestly, you don't have to worry. In fact, worry is your enemy. Anxiety is always the very emotion that gets a fetishist in trouble. Because now you feel stress and what better way to alleviate that stress than to masturbate? But you can't. So now you're more stressed. See how this panic can escalate?

Instead of working yourself up, allow yourself to take in the fetish environment the same way you'd take in a sunset. Enjoy the beauty. Appreciate the aesthetics of your turn-on. There's no reason to feel that you have to act on your fantasies in the moment. Take some mental snapshots that you can enjoy later in the privacy of your own bed. If you have unique, out-of-the-ordinary sexual arousals, consider yourself lucky. Social events that others might find tedious provide hidden enjoyment for you. Just relax and appreciate the uniqueness of you.

Compulsive Behaviors

You might feel that you spend too much time doing research about your fetish online. One fetishist told me that he would often spend hours upon hours on the computer looking for just the right image. Another told me that he'd rather masturbate while surfing the Web than have sex with his wife. Again, these are the very behaviors that members of the psychological community point out when talking about the evils of fetish. They demonstrate the beginnings of compulsive behaviors.

There's a huge difference between exhibiting compulsive behaviors and enjoying your fetish. If you find that your fetish interests are interfering with your work, family and friends, you have to reevaluate your choices. It doesn't mean you have to give up your fetish, you simply have to employ time-management skills and reconsider your priorities. After all, you wouldn't quit your job and hole yourself up in your room to build model trains 24/7, would you? It's the same thing with a fetish.

I'm not suggesting that people who have fetishes never have sexual addictions but I am saying that just because you have a fetish; it doesn't mean that you suffer from sex addiction. Fetish fulfillment and sex addiction do not go hand in hand. They are completely different.

Fetish is a sexual preference you are born with. Addiction is a disorder that must be professionally addressed. If you think you have disordered behavior with your fetish, get some help. However, be wary of the professional who blames your addiction on your fetish. They just don't understand. My advice is to heed their word on addiction but remember that your fetish is yours. You might want to seek out another professional who has a more healthy, organic attitude toward fetish.

In Summary

Fetishistic behavior is only disordered when it is practiced compulsively and used exclusively as a way to self-soothe. Ironically, fetish often becomes out of hand because of guilt factors instilled by others. Humans have a drive to feel accepted and blend into their surroundings. When people are feeling unsupported, unaccepted and secretive, they then develop anxiety. The more the anxiety grows, the more there's a need to self-soothe. And that's when fetishists isolate, spend too much time on fetish websites or engage in risky behaviors. It's usually done out of a wish for acceptance and to dispel debilitating guilt.

Fetish is simply being aroused by something out of the norm. It's not in and of itself a sexual addiction. Fetish behaviors can be managed and controlled. Ideally, we hope that yours will be incorporated into your loving relationship. The more you feel accepted and supported, the less likely you will behave in a disordered, non-consensual way.

And, never forget to love yourself. Be respectful, caring and make sure you get your wishes met in a healthy, balanced and safe way.

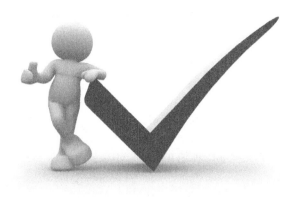

Chapter 22 - Measuring Your Progress: Where Do You Stand Now?

Chapter 3 allowed you to explore your beliefs about fetish. You were given 10 statements expressed by most fetishists and were asked to respond to them. How many of those did you agree with at the time? Let's see how many you agree with now:

Fetish Quiz # 1 – Your Fetish Perception, Reprise:
1. My fetish makes me a freak.
2. My fetish is sick and perverse.
3. I'll keep my fetish a secret until the day I die.
4. I'm not a good person because I have a fetish.
5. I hate that I have a fetish.
6. No woman would want me if they knew what I really desire.
7. It's completely wrong that I think of fetish in order to have an orgasm.
8. Fighting my fetish makes me feel that there's hope for me. Maybe I'll be forgiven on Judgment Day.
9. I'll never accept this part of myself.
10. I'm nothing but an addict.

Fetish Perception Score

Your score should be zero! At this point, I'm sure you know the fallacies of all 10 statements. However, I do want you to be honest. If you're still holding onto some of your old beliefs, it's understandable. These beliefs have been ingrained in you ever since you were young. It's hard to discard them. But please do revisit them.

Ask yourself:
- How is holding onto these beliefs helping me?
- Are these beliefs based on actual fact?
- Do these beliefs help me to be the person I want to be?
- Do these beliefs help me reach my goals?

Keep working. Keep challenging. You'll get there.

An Evolved Fetishist's Perception, Reprise:

In Chapter 3, I also showed you the beliefs of evolved fetishists. Look at them now. How many of these beliefs have you been able to adapt as your own?

Fetish Quiz # 2 – An Evolved Fetishist's Perception, Reprise:

1. My fetish means that I have "out-of-the-box" proclivities.
2. My fetish is a little quirky, but it's just one part of my sexuality.
3. My fetish is sexually based. The only person who ever needs to know is my partner. Even, then, disclosure is solely my choice.
4. I'm a good person based upon my behaviors, interactions and values. Fetish has no bearing on my character.
5. I accept that I have a fetish.
6. I am respectful of the fact that my partner or future partner may not initially understand my fetish. I can make a mindful decision about whether or not I want to tell my partner about my fetish.
7. My thoughts can never hurt anyone. I'm lucky to have something to think about that reliably helps me to orgasm.
8. I don't believe I'll be judged based on my fetish. By accepting myself, I can use my energy to be the best

person I can be.
9. The more I learn, the more I know that I'm okay.
10. I'm in control of my fetish. It doesn't control me.
   I incorporate fetish into my life in a safe, sane, balanced way.

An Evolved Fetishist's Score

I hope you score a 10, which means that you accept every single modified belief. Though they still might seem a bit foreign to you, in time, you'll feel as strongly about these statements as you did about the original ones. It takes a while to internalize a new belief. Keep sticking with it. I know you're well on your way to being an evolved fetishist!

In Summary

The statements given in both fetish quizzes are methods to test your progress. How did you do? Did you notice some internal changes in the way you feel about your fetish?

Progress is something very personal for you. Think about what you'd hoped to accomplish in this program. Only you can decide if you've met your goals.

What was the most important thing you wanted to accomplish? Have you done that? What else would you like to do with your fetish?

I know that many of you just wanted to understand yourselves better. You know, have a different feeling or attitude about your fetish. If you've accomplished this, you've accomplished a great deal.

This program isn't meant to be digested all at once but gradually. Remember, a little goes a long way. Self-acceptance and a rational belief system about fetish is its foundation. You won't be able to have any kind of deep fetish exchange with another person unless you understand and accept your own fetish.

Although it's tempting, don't try to rush in and share your fetish findings with your significant other until you're absolutely ready. That's why it's okay if you only made it through some of the basic tenants. Make sure you accomplish the task laid out in each section until you move on to the next one. It took you many, many years to develop your old belief system. Your current, more-evolved state must be nurtured before you will wholeheartedly be able to fully adopt it as your own.

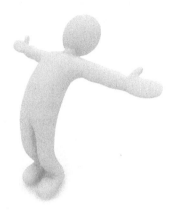

Chapter 23 - Summary/Epilogue

Congratulations! You've taken the journey down the road toward healthy, fetish fulfillment. You've gained education, accomplished self-knowledge and learned effective communication skills. You've also made some important decisions about how to incorporate fetish into your present or future life situation.

You have viable options and the necessary tools for thoughtful decision-making. Acceptance allows for a new, progressive way of thinking about sexuality. Acceptance is key in combating your shame and anxiety.

The cravings belong to you. Accept your fetish as a quirk. Accept it with a sense of humor. Accept it gently. They are yours. You no longer have to feel shame.

You're not making fear-based decisions or buying into a belief system that's not your own. Whatever you decide, you can no longer deny the fact that fetish fulfillment is necessary in order for you to achieve balance and happiness.

Remember that this journey is not linear. It doesn't go from start to finish. It doesn't correlate to reading this book from beginning to end. You are constantly growing and evolving. This is only the start. Be proud of yourself for all that you've accomplished. Thinking rationally will help you in all facets of your life. Real change happens internally. You can travel the globe, buy a house or car and still, your life will be the same. Change occurs only when you allow yourself to experience your own reality with an attitude of acceptance of yourself and loved ones.

This wasn't easy. You had to come to terms with some difficult truths about yourself. Now you have a vision of something different, a new way of thinking and approaching this thing called life. You're well on your way to embodying the existence you were meant to have.

Nothing Has Changed

Many fetishists want to get rid of their fetish. They are supported by society, spouses and even by their therapists. You yourself might have picked up this book thinking it would teach you how to discard your fetish. Sorry if that was your expectation. But I hope you realize that my teachings are giving you a whole lot more. You were rewarded with a new way to view your fetish. I've handed you a belief system that allows you to understand fetish in a positive, rather than a negative, light. Yet, your everyday life is pretty much the same.

Isn't it remarkable? Nothing has changed, yet everything has. You still have the same job, like the same foods and enjoy the same pastimes you always have. Many of you are still in the same relationship, have the same family and live in the same house. You've made absolutely no outer change. The change all occurred within. It's your perception that's changed. And when that inner shift occurs, everything in your world seems different. That's the beauty of real change. It's an inside job.

You may feel different because you're more self-accepting. With self-worth comes confidence. You might be carrying yourself differently or speaking in a more self-assured way. People might notice something has changed but they won't be able to put their finger on it.

Think of it this way: You're still the amazing guy you've always been. Now you're a better version of you, a person who doesn't waste time on societally-imposed judgments. You're a man who makes decisions based on your own thoughts and ideas. Communication comes easily and you can speak your mind without fear of what others think. You can find validity in the opposition but ultimately, you live by your own beliefs. You live your life without apology.

Fetish actualization is a process.

There's no timeframe for absolute sexual actualization. It takes as long as it takes. You're navigating through a sea of "shoulds" imposed upon you by parents, teachers and the public. Right now, you've been exploring. Thinking. Figuring things out. You're writing down your new beliefs and practicing saying them out loud to yourself or your partner. I know that sometimes it doesn't really feel like you. You'll wonder how much you've really changed. But at some point, you'll know because you'll feel it in your body. You'll own the beliefs as much as you professed to believe the original negativity directed toward your triggers.

It will feel spontaneous. You'll know your fetish is okay and you'll never question it again. Sure, you still may be met with opposition but you won't be affected emotionally. You'll be respectful of another person's ideas but you'll also honor your own.

Think of it this way. Imagine if someone told you that they liked vacationing in Canada. You yourself prefer the Caribbean. You'd listen to their ideas but it wouldn't emotionally affect you or make you doubt yourself. The same goes for owning your own beliefs about fetish. Others can have an opinion or conviction. You can listen and understand it. But in the end, you know that your fetish is yours and you choose to accept and enjoy it.

Maybe you already feel the change. If you do, that's awesome. If you don't yet, don't worry, it will come. Keep challenging your old thoughts. When you're feeling shame or guilt, remember to address yourself with compassion and kindness. Never allow yourself to use unkind words or labels. When you find yourself slipping, catch your thoughts before they take over.

Thank You

I have worked with a large number of adult fetishists over the span of my 30-year career as a therapist. I'm always touched by the fact that fetishists are good, honest hardworking people who were dealt an odd set of cards. Not that the cards were bad or wrong, it's just that they're different or quirky. Yet, every fetishist I've ever encountered suffered and berated himself relentlessly. They'd allow the fetish to dictate a life filled with loneliness. They gave the fetish way more power than it deserved.

Life truly is about perception. It's all how we see things. Circumstances don't change. It's all how we choose to view our situation.

I honestly believe that you now have the power to transform the way you view your fetish. No matter what the fetish. No matter how outrageous you think it is. If you accept it, you'll enjoy it. If you accept it, you just might get someone else to accept it, too. Good luck in your journey!

Acknowledgements

Thank you, Vinnie, for being who you are. I love you with all my heart. Without you this book would have never happened. You are the one who gives me the unconditional acceptance to keep going. You are the one human being I can count on and trust. You're also the one that's brought fetish to me as a lifestyle. I think we've proven that fetish is indeed something that grows, evolves and provides enriching experiences.

Thank you, Cathy, for always believing in me and in my work. Without you, I would never have gotten my first projects off the ground. You fought for me and believed in me. Thank you for giving me the opportunity to write and polishing my work into "a shiny diamond," as you so kindly phrased it.

Thank you, Rick, for our weekly talks. I've learned so much from you over the years. You've helped me formulate and validate my own thinking. I've also enjoyed watching you grow tremendously over time. Thank you for your ongoing trust in me.

About The Author

Jackie A. Castro is a licensed Marriage Family Therapist (MFT) with a private practice in Los Angeles, California. She was born and raised in New York City but has lived most of her adult life in California. She studied education and received her BA in Elementary Education from Boston University. She received her Master's Degree in Clinical Psychology from Antioch University and then went on to do post-graduate work at the Institute for Advanced Study of Human Sexuality in San Francisco.

Jackie's gift is being open minded and accepting of all human beings. She is compassionate about their struggles and always maintains an attitude of respect and genuine empathy. She's been actively involved with alternative lifestyle communities for most of her life. Jackie is proud to give voice to a community that's often left unheard.

Jackie currently advocates for those in the fetish community. She also offers individual and couples counseling for all people in need, including, but not limited to, those in the LGBT community, and of course, those who struggle with sexual fetish.

She has written numerous articles, as well as the book *Sex, Fetish and Him* (Volossal Publishing, 2011).

Visit Jackie's website at:
www.therapywithcare.com

Contact her directly at:
therapywithcare@roadrunner.com
or
therapywithcare@gmail.com

CPSIA information can be obtained at www.ICGtesting.com
Printed in the USA
LVOW04s2036060315

429543LV00017B/483/P